The Ikigai Diet
The Secret Japanese Diet to Health and Longevity
Sachiaki Takamiya

# TABLE OF CONTENTS

## Chapter 1 The Secret to Staying Young from the Healthiest People in Japan

## Chapter 6 Low Carb Diet vs. Brown Rice

## Chapter 7 The Superfood Rice Alternatives to Brown Rice

**Chapter 8 Kyodo Ryori: the Authentic Washoku**

**Chapter 9 Wheat vs. Rice: the Ikigai Diet for Europeans**

**Chapter 10 The Seven Foods That Will Age You Faster**

## Chapter 13 Ikigai diet menus

## Chapter 14 Ikigai Exercises

8

# CHAPTER 1

## THE SECRET TO STAYING YOUNG

## FROM THE HEALTHIEST PEOPLE IN JAPAN

# The Way to Stay Young, Healthy, and Happy into Old Age

How many people you know have cancer, diabetes, or dementia? The older you get, the number increases, doesn't it? Having seen people close to you go through these diseases, you now know anyone can develop them. Is it a natural process, and you just have to accept it as you age?

Or is there a way out? What if there was a way not to get sick at all, even in your 80s or 90s? What if you could move around vigorously and continue enjoying your life?

There are people called centenarians who have lived over 100, and many of them continue being active until their final moments. They don't seem to be just disease-free, they seem to be happy and savoring every minute of their life.

What if we could learn from their secrets? In the field of sports or business, it is often said that the best way to acquire skills is to find role models in the field you want to excel at and emulate their strategy. If it is so, we can learn to stay young and healthy by finding role models in the field of wellness and longevity.

Many of these centenarians are in Japan, and Japan is one of the countries with the highest life expectancy. It has mostly had the lowest mortality rate for the last ten years. There are centenarians in other parts of the world, too. Yet, they are usually in small areas, and there aren't many other countries that have such a high concentration of centenarians. In that case, can Japanese people be the role models of health and longevity?

Not all Japanese people are healthy, and not all aspects of Japanese culture are examples of wellness. To learn the Japanese secrets to health and longevity, we need to understand the culture correctly, and we need to find the right crowd, the healthiest people in Japan.

## Are Okinawans Really the Healthiest People in Japan?

Okinawa is known as an island of longevity. In Dan Buettner's book, *The Blue Zones:Lessons for Living Longer From the People Who've Lived the Longest*, he introduced Okinawa as one of the longest-lived regions in the world along with Sardinia in Italy, Nicoya in Costa Rica, Icaria in Greece, and the Seventh-day Adventists community in Loma Linda, California. Okinawa is also featured in the book titled *Ikigai: The Japanese Secret to a Long and Happy Life*, written by Héctor García and Francesc Miralles. It is also well known for the Okinawa Diet, and it's been featured in many TV programs, including Jamie Oliver's cooking program.

## OKINAWA ISN'T RANKED HIGH IN THE NATIONAL LONGEVITY RANKING

In Japan, Okinawans are not necessarily regarded as people of longevity since it was back in the 1980s when Okinawa was ranked high in the national ranking. Recently prefectures like Shiga or Nagano have ranked within the top three and gained the reputation of being long-lived prefectures.

The reason why Okinawa isn't ranked high these days is that the population in the southern part of the island doesn't have as healthy of a lifestyle as they do in the northern part. The southern part has many US military bases and has a strong influence from the American fast-food culture.

Therefore, Okinawa, as a prefecture, isn't regarded as long-lived anymore. Yet, Ogimi village in the northern part, which was featured in *Ikigai: The Japanese Secret to a Long and Happy Life*, is still considered to be one of the longest-lived villages in Japan.

## LONG-LIVED VILLAGES AND SHORT-LIVED VILLAGES OF JAPAN

There was an interesting study done by a doctor in Japan about fifty years ago. Between 1935 and 1971, Dr. Shoji Kondo, a medical professor at Tohoku University and the author of *Nihon No Chojumura Tanmeimura, Long-lived Villages and Short-lived Villages in Japan*, spent 36 years traveling around Japan, visiting 990 villages and towns to investigate the diets of each place. He discovered that there were villages where many residents lived long and villages where many residents didn't live long. He found out that there was a distinct difference between the diets of long-lived villages and short-lived villages.

From Dr. Kondo's research, it isn't clear which place was the longest-lived; he just listed many long-lived places, but Ogimi village was not on the list.

However, in 1974, Hiromich Hagiwara, the co-author of *Long-lived Villages and Short-lived Villages in Japan*, conducted research using Kondo's method and concluded that Ogimi village was the village where people lived the longest that year.

There were many other villages of longevity in Kondo's research. He didn't give specific names, but throughout Japan there were long-lived villages in Kyushu, Shikoku, Sanin, Sanyo, Kinki, Hokuriku, Chubu, Kanto, Tohoku, and Hokkaido. Therefore, spotlighting just Ogimi village and the Okinawan diet doesn't provide a complete picture of Japanese healthy dietary culture.

## DIET MATTERS MORE THAN LOCATION

What is clear from Dr. Kondo's research, though, is the diets of long-lived villages and those of short-lived villages. Ogimi village does have the diet common to long-lived villages.

## DOES LIFESTYLE AFFECT LONGEVITY?

In the book *Ikigai: The Japanese Secret to a Long and Happy Life*, Héctor García and Francesc Miralles give eight factors behind the long lives of the people of Ogimi village.

1. They keep a vegetable garden.

2. They belong to some form of a neighborhood association.

3. They celebrate all the time with music and dance.

4. They have an Ikigai, an important purpose in their life.

5. They are proud of their tradition and local culture.

6. They are passionate about everything they do.

7. They help each other.

8. They are always busy doing something.

The diet is not included here, although they did discuss that the diet contributed to the longevity.

Nonetheless, I discovered something interesting in these eight factors. They apply to Shiga Prefecture and Nagano Prefecture, as well, which are ranked high in the recent longevity ranking.

Since I live in Shiga Prefecture, I have daily encounters with elderly neighbors, and what I have observed so far, six of them apply to my neighbors.

1. They have a garden.

2. They belong to a neighborhood association and have a strong bond with one another: They often chat with one another and are never lonely.

3. They don't necessarily celebrate all the time since we don't have a custom of dancing and singing on the main island of Japan like they do in Okinawa.

4. They have an Ikigai because many of them are both Shintoists and Buddhists, so spirituality plays a big role in their lives.

5. They are proud of their tradition and local culture. People in their seventies aren't anymore, but people in their eighties still retain their pride.

6. They are not necessarily passionate about everything they do.

7. They help each other.

8. They are always busy doing something: They work in the rice field, vegetable field, cutting down trees in the mountains, or fixing their houses.

Therefore apart from the third and the sixth element, they are common among the seniors in rural areas of Shiga Prefecture.

I lived in a rural village in Nagano Prefecture for three years in my teens, and also feel that the six elements seen among my neighbors in Shiga apply to the seniors in Nagano.

I have lived in another rural area of Tochigi Prefecture and observed similar factors among the seniors there, but not in Tokyo where I have also lived. It seems to suggest that those six factors are common characteristics among the senior citizens in the Japanese countryside. Okinawans are unique in that they have a culture of enjoying singing and dancing, as well as having a more joyful personality prevalent among people in a warmer climate. Therefore the third and the sixth are attributes of just Okinawa, but the rest are standard throughout Japan's rural areas.

It means that as far as lifestyle is concerned, the people in Japanese rural communities can be our role models regardless of geographic location.

## DO THEY HAVE SIMILAR DIETS TO OKINAWANS IN THE JAPANESE COUNTRYSIDE?

What about a diet then? Dr. Kondo thinks the diet is the most influential factor in longevity. I already said that Ogimi village had the kind of diet seen among long-lived villages, and I will get into that later. How about other rural areas in Japan? Well, that differs depending on the place. Many of the short-lived villages were also located in the countryside. Being in the country doesn't mean you have a healthy diet. Most villages in Shiga and Nagano were long-lived, according to Dr. Kondo's map, though.

To think of the geographic locations and their diets, we need to take the times into consideration. The situation is very different today from that of the 1960s or '70s. Around that time, the location was relevant, since there were distinct differences among the diets of each region, due to the availability of ingredients. Nevertheless, today most people have access to all kinds of food regardless of where we live. Back then, only some villages had access to fish and seaweed because they were on the coast, but now, we can get seafood everywhere in Japan: Most places are located within a two- to three-hour drive from the coastline in Japan, which makes us one of the biggest fish consuming nations in the world. In the past, many poor villages couldn't afford to buy rice unless they were rice growers, but today, everybody eats rice. In the past, some fishing villages didn't have any space to grow vegetables and ate only rice and fish, but today everybody can eat vegetables. Therefore, today in the rural areas, whether they are fishing villages or rice-growing areas, or mountain regions, they eat regular Washoku, the Japanese food, consisting of rice, seafood, soybeans, and vegetables.

In other words, Washoku today is standard all over Japan, while it varied from place to place in the old days. And standard Washoku is regarded to be one of the core factors in the nation's low mortality rate.

## WHY IS WASHOKU HEALTHY?

Washoku has been registered as a UNESCO Intangible Cultural Heritage of Humanity, for the following characteristics.

1. Diversity and freshness of ingredients, and respect for their inherent flavors.

2. An exceptionally well-balanced and healthy diet.

3. An expression of natural beauty and the changing seasons.

4. Close links with annual events.

One of them is being a well-balanced and healthy diet. In that case, what aspects of Washoku are well-balanced and healthy?

Most meals in Japan have a good balance of carbohydrate-based food, protein-based food, and vitamin-based food, while it isn't the case in some countries. For example, in English speaking countries, you might have eggs and sausages with bread without vegetables for breakfast. In Japan, we have rice, miso soup, pickles, and Natto or eggs. Miso soup usually contains some vegetables, so along with pickles, we get a good portion of vegetables for breakfast. For school lunch, you might have just fried chicken and French fries, without vegetables. Or you might have peanut butter on bread, chips, and an apple or banana. In this case, you have fruit, and therefore you have vitamin-based food, but in my opinion, fruits and vegetables are different in terms of sugar intake. In Japan, school lunches usually consist of rice or bread, soup, a vegetable dish, and a protein-based dish.

It comes from a tradition of Ichiju Sansai, which means one soup three dishes. From Washoku's point of view, each meal should contain rice, soup, pickles, and three side dishes. One of the side dishes is protein-based, such as fish or a soybean-based food. Recently, more people have meat as a protein-based dish. The other two are vegetable-based.

We usually have vegetables in all meals, and we probably eat a lot more vegetables each day than the average people in English speaking countries do.

We don't eat so much sweet. We don't have anything sweet for breakfast, such as cereal with sugar, muffins, or pancakes. We don't have the custom of having dessert after dinner.

Even for our tea breaks, we have green tea with pickles, not with cakes or donuts.

We have a lot of fermented foods such as miso, soy sauce, Natto, and pickles.

We eat a lot of seaweed.

We have a variety of ways to prepare vegetables, such as stewing, steaming, vinegaring, seasoning, and pickling. In the process, we use sesame seeds or vinegar, which are said to have some health benefits.

Generally speaking, we eat much less. That is seen in the amount of each serving at fast food restaurants; you'll be surprised to see how small each portion is when you come to Japan. Our large size coffee is your small size coffee.

Some of you who have been to Japan might disagree with me, thinking Japanese people do eat a lot of sweets and other unhealthy foods.

You are right. That is true. Our diet has changed a lot in recent decades. Many young people and city dwellers now have mixed diets. Many of them have toast for breakfast, and they put butter and jam on it. On weekends, they might even go to a Hawaiian pancake place and have a large portion of pancakes with plenty of cream. They eat at McDonald's, Kentucky Fried Chicken, and Yoshinoya, which is a Japanese fast food restaurant chain serving beef bowls.

Many Japanese dishes are westernized, too. They are called Yoshoku, which means Western food, but they are Japanese-style Western food. A beef bowl is one example. It is a bowl of boiled beef and onions on rice. We didn't have meat at our tables until about a hundred years ago, but now beef, pork, and chicken are served at almost every meal: Buta No Shogayaki, stir-fry pork with ginger; Tonkatsu, deep-fried pork cutlets; Hanbar-gu Teishoku, bunless hamburger platter; and Tori No Karaage, Japanese fried chicken are all typical Japanese dishes now. They are not Washoku, but they are very much part of our dietary culture today, and in many ways, they are more standard than Washoku.

Are they healthy?

They usually come with rice, miso soup, pickles, and salad or other vegetable dishes, which means they still have the format of Ichiju Sansai. Therefore, they are probably more balanced than let's say a hamburger with salad and French fries, or Fried chicken with French fries, or steak with boiled potatoes, carrots, and peas. And yet, I don't think they are good representations of our dietary culture.

On top of that, we have a lot of regular Western dishes, such as pasta, pizza, hamburgers, and steak, as well as other foreign dishes such as ramen and dumplings from China, curry from India, and tacos from Mexico.

Yes, the Japanese dinner table has changed in the last fifty years or so. Most Japanese people have lost touch with the traditional Japanese diet.

This applies mostly to young people and city dwellers but not to seniors in the countryside, at least not to the same degree. The country seniors still predominantly eat Washoku. People in their seventies or younger may eat a lot of Yoshoku, as well, though, but they don't eat regular Western foods like pasta, pizza, and a hamburger.

## ARE ELDERLY PEOPLE IN JAPAN'S RURAL AREAS THE HEALTHIEST IN JAPAN?

That means senior citizens in the countryside are the people who still retain our traditional diet, and have a lifestyle similar to the one in Ogimi village. Does it mean they are the healthiest people in Japan now?

To answer this question, we need to look at the diets that long-lived villages had and the diets short-lived villages had during Dr. Kondo's discovery.

## THE DIET OF LONG-LIVED VILLAGES

The people in long-lived villages had a lot of soybeans, vegetables, especially green and yellow vegetables, and seaweed. That is the same at most dinner tables in the Japanese countryside today. Even places where they previously couldn't get hold of some of these ingredients are now able to obtain them.

## THE DIET OF SHORT-LIVED VILLAGES

On the other hand, people in short-lived villages had a lot of white rice and didn't have enough vegetables, soybeans, and seaweed. Yes, white rice was the problem. According to Dr. Kondo, eating a lot of white rice was the core factor of people living short. He discovered, after checking the diets of 990 villages and towns all over Japan from Hokkaido to Okinawa, that people in short-lived villages and towns were all eating a lot of white rice without exception. It is quite surprising because white rice is our staple food, and that is the main dish in Washoku. It is very much part of our culture, and we are supposed to be healthy.

Apparently, people in Shiga didn't eat a lot of white rice; we ate Mugimeshi, rice with barley, instead. It was a common custom in many parts of Japan because rice was a luxury. Only the wealthy and rice growers ate rice. Even for rice growers, rice was their commodity, and some of them ate other grains at home.

Another doctor called Tsuneo Matsuike hypothesized that Mugimeshi was one of the causes behind the people of Shiga's longevity in his book *Nihonichi No Chojuken To Sekaiichi No Chojumura No Cho Ni Ii Shokuji, The Gut-Friendly Diets of Japan's Number One Longevity Prefecture and The World's Number One Longevity Village.*

In Ogimi village, they eat a lot of sweet potatoes as their staple instead of white rice.

The fact that we got wealthier and are able to afford rice turned out to be unfortunate. Our diet got worse than that of long-lived villages. Yet, our diet is probably better than that of short-lived villages since we eat white rice, soybeans, vegetables, seaweed, fish, and some meat, while some people in short-lived villages had a lot of white rice with just a small amount of salty pickles, no other vegetables or seaweed. Or they had fish with a lot of white rice. Modern-day country Washoku is more balanced.

Nevertheless, I don't think I can say that seniors in the countryside are the healthiest people in Japan because they also eat regular vegetables instead of organic vegetables, and they use regular seasonings, which have food additives instead of natural ones. Yes, they eat Washoku, but the quality of Washoku isn't as good as before because the ingredients are not natural anymore. It is a problem throughout all of Japanese society; our diet is not natural and healthy, whether it is in the cities or the countrysides.

The older generations in the rural areas retain the traditional lifestyle to a certain degree, but a lot of the good essence has been lost, unfortunately. They had an organic diet when they were younger, but they can no longer have access to foods with pure natural ingredients since our way of food production has changed. And yet they don't try to do anything about it. They are not health conscious people.

That is the bottom line. I cannot say they are the healthiest and should be our role models because of their mentality. They happen to be well because they just followed their tradition, which happens to be good. Nonetheless, when the social norms changed to be using agricultural chemicals or composts of cattle eating genetically modified corns, or fertilizers contaminated by radiation, they also changed by continuing to follow it without question. Their diet when they were younger is still good for us to model, but their mentality isn't.

I don't know about the seniors in Ogimi village because I have not been there, but this is the impression I get from the seniors in Shiga, Nagano, and Tochigi. I don't think it is a regional thing; it is probably the same throughout Japan.

## SHIZENHA, OUR LAST HOPE?

Does this mean we don't have healthy people left in Japan anymore? Young people have been modernized, and so have the city dwellers. Country senior citizens were the only hope left, but they, too, seem to have lost the authentic Washoku diet.

Well, there is our last hope. There is a growing population of young people called Shizenha, which means naturalists, and they eat radiation-free organic food, brown rice, macrobiotic food, and fermented food.

They have inherited the traditional diet from their grandparents' generations, and they practice it in its original form, so in many ways, they have the authentic Japanese diet.

On top of that, they have the scientific understanding to evaluate their diet. They don't just follow it because it was the traditional way; they experiment to see if the diet actually works. Some older generations in the long-lived areas still retain their traditional natural diet, but I don't think they have the scientific knowledge to back up their wisdom.

Many of these young, naturally conscious people have moved to the countryside from cities and lead sustainable ways of living. They grow rice and vegetables using organic farming, natural farming, and permaculture.

## THE LITTLE KNOWN JAPANESE NATURAL PHILOSOPHY

They also studied Japanese natural philosophy, which wasn't shared among the members of the general public so much, including seniors in long-lived areas. It is central to most Japanese martial arts; healing arts such as Shiatsu or acupuncture; Zen; and the macrobiotic diet. It was influenced by Chinese medicine, and it has a holistic understanding of wellness. Although the entire Japanese culture was influenced by it in one way or another, it has been an esoteric side of Japanese culture, and you had to seek to gain the knowledge.

## HOW NATURALISTS ARE UPGRADING JAPANESE NATURAL PHILOSOPHY

The fact that the naturalists study Japanese natural philosophy separates them from centenarians in long-lived villages; they are seekers while centenarians weren't.

How about Zen monks and masters of martial arts or healing arts? There must be centenarians among them.

The masters of the Japanese natural philosophy are the older generation, too, and they tend to hold a more rigid structure. Some of the principles in Japanese natural philosophy aren't relevant in modern times.

Those naturalists, however, are young people who are flexible enough to break away from the rigid structure of tradition and to incorporate modern approaches into their practice.

They are making an unprecedented breakthrough in our culture, restoring the old wisdom and polishing it with the energy of Indigo and Crystal generations. Through this, they are releasing the truly authentic wisdom, which had been hidden under the rigid structure.

In my opinion, they are the healthiest people in Japan.

## JAPANESE SHIZENHA: ROLE MODELS OF HEALTH

When you model someone for health and longevity, it is vital to emulate not only their diet and lifestyle, but also their mentality. Japanese senior citizens in longevity areas can be our role models for their diets and lifestyles when they were younger, but when it comes to their mentality, it is best not to follow them. The Japanese Shizenha people, however, can be our role models in all these areas.

The *Ikigai Diet* I am going to introduce here is the diet, lifestyle, and mentality of these Shizenha people.

Earlier, I mentioned that Shizenha people ate macrobiotic food, and they studied Japanese natural philosophy, by which the macrobiotic diet was influenced. In that case, is the Ikigai Diet any different from the macrobiotic diet?

## THE IKIGAI DIET VS. THE MACROBIOTIC DIET

Some Shizenha people practice the macrobiotic diet, and the macrobiotic way of eating is popular in Japan, as well. However, that is not the only diet we have in Japan. Like many people associate Okinawa as the place of longevity, some of you might associate Japanese natural food culture with the macrobiotic diet. There are great elements in the macrobiotic diet that we can learn from, but at the same time, its rather strict principles tend to exclude some components within the Washoku culture, which I think are relevant to our wellness and longevity.

There are other newer popular diets in Japan, such as Miraishoku Tsubutsubu, Nagaokashiki Kosogenmai, and Banno Koboeki. The macrobiotic diet isn't the only option, and Shizenha people select what works for them from a wide variety of choices.

The Ikigai Diet doesn't have a specific principle such as Yin and Yang; it is a diet that I composed based on my observations of Shizenha people and my own experience of leading a natural lifestyle.

## AGING 21 YEARS YOUNGER

I am not a doctor nor a nutritionist; nothing I write in this book guarantees a medical effect. I am just presenting my observations and experiences. I am in my late fifties now, but I haven't had any problems at my medical checkups so far. People tell me that I generally look much younger, and I was diagnosed that my vascular age was twenty-one years younger.

I am one of the Shizenha people, and I practice the very lifestyle I am talking about here. I have personal experiences in trying different diets, and finally settled on this diet. I have studied recent scientific discoveries in the field of gut health and longevity, and have incorporated them into this diet.

## MORE THAN A DIET; A WAY TO TRANSFORM SOCIETY

I think the Ikigai Diet is the most cutting edge diet of Japanese natural food culture because it isn't just good for your health, it makes you happier and helps you live with Ikigai, a purpose you need for your happiness. This connection of diet and mentality is crucial since our gut health is influenced by both areas. Instead of having medical or nutritional expertise, I have been a philosophical seeker all my life, searching for ways of personal and social happiness. That makes me able to bring more holistic elements to the diet. Along with Ikigai, I am incorporating a 300-year-old philosophical concept from Shiga Prefecture called Sanpo-Yoshi into this diet. Sanpo-Yoshi is a way to transform society where everybody is happy.

# CHAPTER 2

## IKIGAI AND SANPO-YOSHI

## WHAT IS IKIGAI?

Ikigai means something you have or do that is worth living for, that is rewarding or fulfilling. It is often interpreted as a small joy in your daily life. You can find Ikigai in almost anything as long as you feel joy and meaning in that activity. You can feel Ikigai when you jog in the morning, you can feel Ikigai when you play with your children, and you can feel Ikigai when you are immersed in work you love.

People might ask you, "what is your Ikigai?" And you might answer, "My morning jog is my Ikigai," "My children are my Ikigai," or "My work is my Ikigai."

Therefore, for most Japanese people, it isn't a big deal; it doesn't have a deep philosophical meaning like it is thought to be in the West. The way the word Ikigai is interpreted in other countries is a little exaggerated. I don't think it is even considered to be a factor of longevity in Japan. We all have Ikigai in one way or another, and having Ikigai doesn't separate us from the rest of the population.

Having said that, there is another meaning to the word Ikigai. It means your life purpose or reason for living.

If you are a philosophical person, you might give a deeper answer to the same question: What is your Ikigai?

"Bringing justice to the world is my Ikigai," "improving the educational system is my Ikigai," or "helping people to be happy is my Ikigai."

In this book, I am interpreting Ikigai as a life purpose or a life mission, and if I contemplate the meaning, we need to go beyond our subjective feeling of enjoyment or fulfillment. We need to understand the structure of society, and expand our consciousness to feel what happiness really is. Can your work be Ikigai if your company makes profits by exploiting others even though it is satisfying to you? Can your hobby be Ikigai when you enjoy it so much that you prioritize it over your family? What really is happiness for us? What is our purpose in life? The Ikigai I am talking about here isn't just rewarding to you, but it is also satisfying to your family and people around you, and gratifying to society. In other words, for Ikigai to give justice to its true meaning, it needs to have the element of Sanpo-Yoshi.

## WHAT IS SANPO-YOSHI?

Sanpo-Yoshi is a philosophy of Omi-merchants from Shiga Prefecture who were considered to be the most successful merchants in Japan from the medieval period to the 18th century. This philosophy stated that every business the Omi-merchants conducted needed to be beneficial to the seller, the buyer, and society in general. In short, a business must result in a three-way satisfaction.

Sanpo means three directions, and Yoshi means good or happy, and Sanpo-Yoshi contains three Yoshi.

**Urite-Yoshi:** This means the seller is happy
**Kaite-Yoshi:** This means the buyer is happy
**Seken-Yoshi:** This means society is happy.

This is a concept in business, but we can apply it in other fields, too. For example, in the Ikigai Diet, we apply it in pursuit of happiness.

**Jibun-Yoshi**: I am happy
**Aite-Yoshi**: You are happy
**Seken-Yoshi**: Society is happy.

You, in this case, means people whom you have direct contacts with, such as your family, friends, and coworkers. When you feel Ikigai, it is better to feel it in an activity which doesn't just make you happy, but also makes your family happy. For example, instead of feeling your Ikigai in playing golf, which either you do alone or with your business associates, you can feel your Ikigai in going for walks with your family. In this way, you can feel happy and so can your family. It also makes society happy since it is environmentally friendlier than playing golf on a golf course, which was probably built by destroying a forest.

Another example is that instead of finding your Ikigai in your work and giving 100% of your time and energy to it, you can find your Ikigai in the work-style that includes time for your family.

Or, instead of finding your Ikigai in winning a business competition, you can find your Ikigai by coming up with ways to make doing business profitable for all involved.

This applies to diet, too. By eating delicious food, you can make yourself happy so that it can be Jibun-Yoshi, but it may not make others happy. Therefore, it may not be Aite-Yoshi. On the other hand, if you eat natural food, it makes you healthy and happy. Usually, it makes people around you healthy and happy, as well, because what you eat influences your family and friends. If you cook a healthy meal and invite your friends over, your friends can become interested in how you cook. By eating well, you will be mentally and physically in balance, and you will be a positive person to be around with. Therefore, it can be Aite-Yoshi, too.

## WHAT IS A SOCIALLY FRIENDLY DIET?

What about Seken-Yoshi, then? Can eating natural food be good for society? The food we eat is related to the way we produce food, and the way we grow food influences the environment and our social structure. So, what we eat affects society. By eating organically grown food or naturally grown food, you can support organic farming or natural farming, both of which are better for our environment. Therefore, eating natural food can be Seken-Yoshi, as well. Another thing you want to pay attention to is to eat locally grown food. By eating locally, you are helping to reduce our energy consumption to transport food.

Both organic and local food production help fight against climate change, and therefore they can help you live longer. After all, what is the point of extending your lifespan if your life is at risk by natural disasters? Personal health and global health are related, and a path toward longevity should include social change.

Thus, eating locally grown natural food can be a Sanpo-Yoshi diet. Nonetheless, natural food is a vague term; there are different kinds of natural foods: Vegetarian cheeseburgers and quiches are categorized as natural food, and so are pickled daikon and miso soup. Does simply using organic or non-animal ingredients make the food natural?

In the following chapters, I will illustrate more in detail about what you can eat and how to eat based on the diet of Shizenha, Japanese naturalists.

# CHAPTER 3

# ORGANICALLY GROWN VEGETABLES VS. NATURALLY GROWN VEGETABLES

## Regular Washoku vs. Shizenha Washoku

Whether you eat Washoku or Western food, the ingredients you use matter. Japanese naturalists cook Washoku using natural ingredients, which makes their Washoku different from regular Washoku. Washoku served at most restaurants in Japan are not made from organically grown ingredients. In fact, if you ask waiters or waitresses at restaurants whether they use organic ingredients or not, they are most likely unable to answer your questions right away; in some cases they won't even know. Japan is the least conscious country within the advanced countries regarding food traceability.

Therefore, when you come to Japan, it is better to eat home-cooked meals at people's houses or natural food restaurants. There aren't as many natural food restaurants as there are in the West, but the number is increasing as the number of naturally conscious people is growing.

Now let me talk about what you can do in your home country, since most of you are reading this book in different parts of the world. There is so much you can do with your own food culture by choosing the right ingredients. The first step is using organically grown ingredients or naturally grown ingredients as much as possible, which include grains such as rice and wheat, vegetables, beans, oil, seasonings like miso, salt, and soy sauce.

## What are Naturally Grown Ingredients?

When I say naturally grown ingredients, I am talking about food grown using what is called Natural Farming. Natural Farming is a method of farming that was developed by Masanobu Fukuoka, the author of *The One-Straw Revolution*, or Yoshikazu Kawaguchi, where you don't till the land, you don't use fertilizers (not even organic ones), and you only do a limited amount of weeding. The reason why you don't till the earth is that the tilling will destroy the microorganisms inside the soil, which can help vegetables grow. So, by not tilling, you let the microorganism take care of the vegetables, and you don't need to add fertilizers. You don't cut every weed, because by having some weeds left, insects don't concentrate on the vegetables. In the same vein, you don't kill every bug, because some bugs are natural predators of other insects and they can protect the vegetables from them. Also, in Natural Farming, you don't water the plants; you let the rain take care of it.

Organic farming sometimes uses too much fertilizer, and it creates oversized vegetables. By intervening in the natural process too much, you weaken the plants, making them susceptible to disease. In Natural Farming, however, the vegetables are more balanced, absorbing only what was available in nature at the time. No one has said it, and it is just my feeling, but maybe it has the same effect as fasting on humans. By going through some hungry period, vegetables can be in their ideal state.

Having said that, Natural Farming is more difficult to put into practice for commercial farmers; it is more suitable for people leading self-sufficient lifestyles. Therefore, you don't see many naturally grown products on the market. If you want to obtain them, you may have to grow your own.

To find out more about Natural Farming, you can click the link below.
*Japanese Natural Farming Guru Kawaguchi Yoshikazu*
https://www.nippon.com/en/people/e00120/

**GROWING YOUR OWN FOOD IS A NEW DIETARY CULTURE OF JAPAN**

Growing your own food is actually better for your health: It is the most local food you can access: By working in the soil, you can contact all kinds of bacteria which benefit your overall well-being: You become more aligned with natural rhythms such as seasons and weather: The fact that most centenarians live in the countryside and work in the fields might suggest that the natural living found in the countryside is the key. When we talk about diet, we need to look at it holistically, and changing your diet means changing your whole lifestyle, not just what you eat.

Growing your own food isn't a dietary method, but people who practice it produce a natural diet based on their farming lifestyle, and therefore we can say it is another dietary culture. They eat what they have in their garden. Unlike the practitioners of other diets, they don't select ingredients based on their health benefits but what they can grow and harvest. Their lifestyle comes before their diet. This movement is growing in Japan, and many Shizenha people follow it.

Natural Farming isn't widely practiced in the West, and biodynamic farming is more common. Biodynamically grown ingredients are also good, so if that's what's available to you, that's fine. Use whatever is accessible in your region.

Yes, ingredients do count, but they alone don't make your food natural, there are ways of preparing food that can help you gain natural energy effectively, and that is one of the secrets of Washoku.

# CHAPTER 4

# HOW TO OPTIMIZE FERMENTED FOODS TO ACTIVATE AUTOPHAGY

## Eating Washoku with Natural Ingredients Adds Wings to a Tiger

As far as organic ingredients are concerned, you already have a great environment in the West. Organic foods are widely available. You can even buy them in many supermarkets now. The next step is to learn how to prepare foods that can give you further health benefits. The traditional Japanese diet has a lot to offer in this field. And yet, you don't need to follow strict recipes; you can grasp the essence of them and apply it to your own dishes.

### Fermented Foods and Gut Health

One of the essences of Washoku is using a lot of fermented food: We use miso, soy sauce, Mirin sweet sake in our everyday cooking. We eat Natto, fermented soybeans, and many different kinds of pickles regularly.

Fermented foods are considered to nurture our health in Japan; they benefit intestinal bacteria. Recently, many Western doctors such as Justin and Erica Sonnenburg, the authors of *The Good Gut: Taking Control of Your Weight, Your Mood, and Your Long-term Health,* have begun to recognize the importance of microbiota and intestines for our well-being and longevity.

In oriental medicine, your organs are critical. They relate to certain emotions that can be adjusted to improve your mental state. In Japanese traditional medicine, the intestines are essential and are regarded as the second brain. The intestines are located in the belly area that the Japanese people know as Hara. The place is so significant that it is central to all martial arts like karate and Aikido, as well as Shiatsu, a natural healing method. We move from Hara and feel Ki energy, which radiates from Hara. In Zen meditation, we breathe through Hara.

In their book *The Good Gut: Taking Control of Your Weight, Your Mood, and Your Long-term Health,* Dr. Justin and Erica Sonnenburg say that fermented foods are one of the gut-friendly foods, and they foster our healthy gut microbiota.

## FERMENTED FOODS AND AUTOPHAGY

Fermented foods such as miso, soy sauce, and Natto contain a polyamine called spermidine which activates autophagy, a cellular recycling process, according to Dr. Tamotsu Yoshimori, who was a co-researcher of Dr. Yoshinori Ohsumi, the 2016 Nobel Prize winner in Physiology or Medicine, by discovering the mechanism of autophagy. Dr. Tamotsu Yoshimori is the author of *Life Science Nagaikisezaruwoenaijidai No Seimeikagakukogi. Life Science: A Life Science Lecture for the Age When We All Have to Live Long.* The book is currently a number 1 best seller on Amazon in Japan. Autophagy is in the spotlight now as one of the most significant mechanisms of longevity, and methods such as intermittent fasting and high-intensity interval training are gaining popularity since they are said to boost this cellular regenerating function. And now fermented foods are in the limelight, too.

## AN AUTOPHAGY ACTIVATING SUPERFOOD: NATTO

Natto contains the highest amount of spermidine, the autophagy activating polyamine, among the three fermented foods I mentioned earlier. It contains 56.1 micrograms per gram, while miso containing 14.4 mcg/g, and soy sauce containing 12.1 mcg/g. I consider Natto to be the king of fermented foods and the most superior superfood. Natto germ, whose official name is Bacillus subtilis, is considered to be the strongest germ, and it doesn't die even when it is boiled at 100-degrees Celsius (212 Fahrenheit). Natto is also known for containing a high amount of vitamin K2 and 5-ALA, both of which are said to protect us from infectious diseases.

Natto was recognized as the number one food in a vote of the top 10 healthiest foods, determined by 300 doctors in Japan in January 2019.

The followings are the reasons why Natto was selected to be the healthiest.

1. It improves the condition of our intestinal environment.
2. It prevents cerebral infarctions and cardiac infarctions.
3. It prevents arteriosclerosis.
4. It prevents type 2 diabetes.
5. It prevents cancer.
6. It prevents dementia.

I haven't heard of any negative comments about Natto, and I haven't come across any other food that has such a high reputation.

Natto has a pungent smell, a strong taste, and sticky texture, making it an acquired taste. Some people love it, and others hate it. I would say about half of the Japanese people like it, which is quite a high number, compared to other superfoods like Goya, an Okinawan vegetable that has a bitter taste. Among foreign people, Natto isn't so popular, but I know many Westerners who love it.

There are a variety of ways to eat Natto, if you don't like the regular way of eating it, which is to eat it with spring onions, mustard, and soy sauce: You can put Natto in a pasta dish, you can put it in curry, and you can put it on pizza, as well.

I have some recipes on my blog.
https://ikigaidiet.com/category/natto-recipe/

You can buy Natto in many places now, including Japanese grocery stores and natural food stores.

If you can't find Natto in your area, you can always make it. One good thing about Natto is that it isn't difficult to make. To make miso, it takes 8 to 10 months, but it takes only 72 hours to make Natto.

I have step by step instructions in my blog.
*How to Make Natto from Rice Straw Sticks*
http://ikigaidiet.com/how-to-make-natto-from-rice-straw-sticks/

I recommend that you make fermented foods at home anyway. Most pickles are easy to make. Pickled daikon and pickled Chinese cabbage are common in Japan, but you can make pickles from almost any vegetable. Use whatever you have at home and whatever you can grow in your garden.

The easiest way of making pickles is pickling vegetables with sea salt and filtered water. It will bring out the lactic acid bacteria from the vegetables and ferment them. You can make them in a few days.

You can find tons of YouTube videos on how to make pickles.

## THE 60 KILOGRAM RICE BAG CARRYING WOMEN OF THE PAST

It is good to ferment food at home so that you can release good bacteria in your house. What was significant about Japanese people in the past was that they didn't just eat fermented food on a regular basis, they made fermented food at home, and they were constantly surrounded by these effective bacteria. Unfortunately, those helpful bacteria have vanished from our homes now due to the decreasing number of households making fermented foods and the spread of germicides. Japanese people used to be vigorous. It was common for women to carry 60 kilograms (132 pounds) of rice; I once saw a picture of a woman carrying three bags of rice weighing 180 kilograms (397 pounds) at a rice carrying competition. Young Shizenha, Japanese naturalists, are bringing back this tradition, and it is becoming a new trend to make miso, pickles, and Natto at home.

## LOCAL BACTERIA VS. COMMERCIALLY PRODUCED BACTERIA

One advantage of making fermented food at home is you can use local bacteria. It is better to use bacteria from the land you live in; they are the most suitable to your body. For example, if you make Natto with rice straw from a local farm, preferably organic, you will be absorbing your regional Natto germs, and it matches you more than commercially produced Natto with bacilli of unknown places.

Now you know that Shizenha people eat organically and naturally grown foods and fermented foods, what else do we do when we eat? In the next chapter, I will share with you some concepts from Zen Shojin diet and current health trends.

# CHAPTER 5

## ZEN SHOJIN DIET

## ICHIBUTSU ZENTAI SHOKU

We have a concept called Ichibutsu Zentai Shoku in Japanese natural food culture. It means to eat food as a whole. When you eat rice, it is better to eat brown rice because it is in its original form and is in the most balanced state. When you eat bread, it is preferable to eat whole wheat bread to white bread. When you eat fish, it is more advisable to eat small fish because you can eat the whole thing instead of eating just one part of a large fish. When you eat a vegetable like a carrot, it is more nutritious to eat the whole carrot without peeling the skin because the skin contains much of the dietary fiber, and it is a waste to throw it away.

It is a Buddhist concept and initially found in Shojin Ryori, which means Shojin cooking or Shojin diet. Shojin Ryori was practiced among monks in Zen monasteries for over 700 years since the Kamakura Period. It was first advocated outside of the Zen community at the beginning of the 20th century by Sagen Ishizuka, who started a natural food group called Shokuyokai. Since then, it has become a part of Japanese natural food culture. George Ohsawa, the founder of the macrobiotic diet, was a member of Shokuyokai, and he incorporated this concept into his diet. Therefore, Ichibutsu Zentai Shoku is a macrobiotic concept as well.

It is popular among Shizenha people, and in the Ikigai Diet, we value it, too.

Do you remember the research conducted by Dr. Shoji Kondo that I referenced in Chapter 1? Dr. Kondo is the author of *Nihon No Chojumura Tanmeimura, Long-lived Villages and Short-lived Villages in Japan.* He spent 36 years traveling around Japan, visiting 990 villages and towns to investigate the diets of each place. He discovered that there were villages where many residents lived long and villages where many residents didn't live long. He found out that there was a distinct difference between the diets of long-lived villages and short-lived villages.

The interesting thing is that people in long-lived villages mostly ate small fish. People who were eating a part of big fish were all short-lived. I don't think they were practicing Ichibutsu Zentai Shoku; they happened to eat small fish because big fish was a luxury.

## SHINDOFUJI

Shindofuji is another concept in Shojin Ryori, and later advocated by Sagen Ishizuka—eating what is grown locally and what is harvested in season.

Eating locally grown food is beneficial for your health as well as for the environment. This is because locally grown vegetables were helped by bacteria living in your land, and local bacteria are the most suitable to your body, as I said in the section of fermenting at home.

When you grow your own food, which I highly recommend, you start eating what you can harvest each season, so you naturally start eating according to Shindofuji. Choosing what vegetables to put into your miso soup and vegetable dishes will be easy: Use what you can harvest that day.

Among people who practice the raw food diet, I sometimes see them eating a lot of tropical fruit on their YouTube videos. If you live in a tropical zone, that is okay, but if you live in a temperate zone, it isn't Shindofuji since you can't grow those types of fruit in your region.

Among vegan people, too, I sometimes see people drinking almond milk or coconut milk, and if almonds and coconuts are imported from faraway places, it isn't Shindofuji either.

I don't mean to say you shouldn't eat them because of that. Maybe there are other elements to consider, and you want to juggle them around to decide your priority. I just wanted to point out that this is another element to consider.

## MA GO WA YA SA SHI I, THE BUZZWORD IN THE JAPANESE NATURAL FOOD COMMUNITY

Ma Go Wa Ya Sa Shi I is not a concept from Shojin Ryori, but it is popular now among Shizenha people. Ma Go Wa Ya Sa Shi I means your grandchildren are kind. It is used as a mnemonic device to remember what foods to eat daily. It is advocated by a food researcher and doctor called Hiroyuki Yoshimura to spread the benefits of Washoku.

Ma stands for Mame, which means beans.

Go stands for Goma, which means Sesame seeds.
Wa stands for Wakame seaweed.
Ya stands for Yasai, which means vegetables.
Sa stands for Sakana, which means fish.
Shi stands for Shitake mushrooms.
I stands for Imo, which means potatoes, including sweet potatoes and taros.

Ma Go Wa Ya Sa Shi I is a guideline to promote the healthy aspects of Washoku culture. You hear about it all the time, almost at every healthy eating seminar you attend. It is a buzzword in the Japanese natural food community.

If I were to translate it into English, it would be something like BSSVFMP.

B: beans
S: Seeds such as sesame seeds, nuts such as almonds
S: Seaweed such as Wakame, Hijiki, Konbu, and Nori
V: Vegetables
F: Fish
M: Mushrooms
P: Potatoes, sweet potatoes, taros

It is a great guideline for creating the balance seen in Washoku in your daily meal. I recommend you use Ma Go Wa Ya Sa Shi I as much as possible in preparing your daily meals. You don't have to have all of them in each meal, but try to have as many as you can in a day or in a week.

As for fish, you don't have to have it a lot. It is common in Washoku because we are an island nation surrounded by the sea. In the Ikigai Diet, I recommend that you eat fish occasionally, and when you do, you eat small fish as in Ichibutsu Zentai Shoku. Small fish is better from the food chain point of view, too: It has fewer heavy metals.

It is also safer to eat wild caught fish, not farmed fish, since farmed fish contains antibiotics.

If you are a vegetarian or vegan, you don't want to eat fish at all, then you don't need to. I sometimes eat blue skinned fish such as mackerel or sardine because they contain omega-3 fatty acids called EPA and DHA, which are difficult to get from plant-based food. The fact that many centenarians include fish in their diets might suggest that it is better to eat fish sometimes for a nutritional aspect, depending on how you are obtaining omega-3 fatty acids.

Anyway, Ma Go Wa Ya Sa Shi I are similar to the diets of long-lived villages identified by Dr. Kondo; they ate a lot of beans, vegetables, seaweed, and potatoes, especially sweet potatoes. Sweet potatoes were staple foods in many long-lived villages, including Ogimi Village in Okinawa. It looks like you'll be in good shape if you eat Ma Go Wa Ya Sa Shi I.

What about grains? Ma Go Wa Ya Sa Shi I don't include grains, do they? That is strange, considering rice is a staple food in Washoku. I'll talk about it later since it involves carbs.

### THE FIBER RICH FOODS OF MA GO WA YA SA SHI I

Dietary fiber is another element you want to look into when you want to be healthy. Justin and Erica Sonnenburg consider it to be the core for your gut-microbiota. A fiber diet feeds and makes good intestinal bacteria thrive.

Dr. Yoshimi Benno, the author of *Hyakusaimade Genkinahito Wa Nani Wo Tabeteiruka, What Do People Who Are Active Until 100 Years Old Eat?* also says dietary fiber is the key to your gut health. He has taken stool samples of many centenarians and came to that conclusion.

Foods that contain dietary fiber are whole grains such as brown rice, barley, and oats; beans such as soybeans, lentils, and kidney beans; vegetables such as carrots, daikon radishes, squashes, broccoli, and burdocks; potatoes such as sweet potatoes and taros; seaweed such as wakame and hijiki; seeds and nuts such as sesame seeds, pumpkin seeds, almond nuts, and peanuts.

Looking at the list, many of them are part of Ma Go Wa Ya Sa Shi I. That means if you eat Ma Go Wa Ya Sa Shi I or BSSVFMP, you get plenty of dietary fiber.

It is also notable that carrots and squashes are on the list of high fiber foods because these green yellow vegetables were especially eaten a lot in long-lived villages where Dr. Kondo visited. This reinforces the fact that dietary fiber is the key to our long life.

## ICHIJU SANSAI: ONE SOUP THREE DISHES

As I mentioned in Chapter 1, the standard way of eating Washoku is Ichiju Sansai, which means rice, soup, pickles, and three small dishes. One of the reasons why Washoku is healthy is it has the tradition of Ichiju Sansai to make every meal well-balanced. It has a good balance of carbohydrate-based food, vitamin-based food, and protein-based food.

I was very surprised when I first went to Australia and had breakfast with just bread, eggs, and sausages. I had never seen a meal without vegetables before that. Later in my life, I learned that only French fries and fried chicken were served for school lunch at some schools in the United States. In Japan, we always have vegetables in every meal, and that applies to school lunch, too, because of the custom of Ichiju Sansai.

So, the idea of Ichiju Sansai is to create a well-balanced meal, and it doesn't matter whether you have two or four side dishes instead of three dishes as long as you have the complete meal. For side dishes, we might have grilled fish as dish 1, cold tofu as dish 2, and stewed, steamed, vinegared, or seasoned vegetables as dish 3. We always have soup, though, since Ichiju means one soup, and soup has a function of warming up our body, which helps boost our immune system. We usually have miso soup as a soup dish, which gives a further benefit as a fermented food. We always have rice and pickles, too. A dish of pickles is not considered as a side dish.

## NIMONO, SUNOMONO, AND AEMONO

Typical Washoku cooking styles are Nimono, stewed vegetables; Sunomono, vinegared vegetables; and Aemono, seasoned vegetables.

A popular Nimono dish is stewed carrots, burdocks, Shiitake mushrooms, and Satoimo, taro. You stew them with soy sauce, brown sugar or raw sugar, mirin, and a small amount of sake.

A popular Sunomono dish is vinegared cucumbers and wakame seaweed. Vinegar is said to slow down the rising of the blood sugar level, so having some sort of Sunomono dish in each meal is a good idea.
A popular Aemono dish is seasoned spinach with sesame seeds. You put spinach in boiling water for about one minute. Then you cool it with cold

water and squeeze it to dehydrate it. You sprinkle sesame seeds over it and add soy sauce.

If you have those Nimono, Sunomono, and Aemono dishes, you are already covering taros, Shitake, wakame, and sesame seeds from Ma Go Wa Ya Sa Shi I.

## IDEAL ICHIJU SANSAI DINNER

From the Ikigai Diet's point of view, here is what I recommend as an ideal dinner.

Rice: Brown rice
Soup: Miso soup with seaweed, seasonal vegetables, and tofu.
Pickles: Pickled seasonal vegetables
Dish 1: Natto
Dish 2: Boiled or steamed leafy vegetables with sesame seeds or nuts (Aemono)
Dish 3: Stewed or steamed or cooked root vegetables (Nimono)

You don't always have to have three dishes; two is okay, and sometimes one is enough. For lunch, you can have brown rice, miso soup, and pickles: No side dishes. For breakfast, either you skip it or have just brown rice and miso soup.

If you are doing a low carb diet, you might be wondering why I am recommending brown rice as part of Ichiju Sansai meal. I am familiar with the concept of reducing one's carbohydrate intake, and I don't entirely disagree with it. As I said before, I am not a doctor, nor a nutritionist; nothing I write in this book guarantees a medical effect. I am just presenting dietary practices of one of the healthiest people in the world, but it doesn't mean it works for everybody. Since we all have different physical makeups and live in different environments, just because it works for some people doesn't always mean it works for others, too. If you have diabetes, for example, you have a different approach from someone who doesn't have any chronic conditions. For people with chronic diseases, I suggest that you consult your doctor first. For healthy individuals, I recommend brown rice, and I will explain why in the next chapter.

# CHAPTER 6

# LOW CARB DIET VS. BROWN RICE

## SHORT-TERM DIET VS. LONG-TERM DIET

I think there are two kinds of diet; the ones that serve as temporary measures for certain conditions, and the others which are more long-term eating habits. Low carb diets that suggest you should avoid carbohydrates entirely can show some results if you do it for a certain period, for diabetes or losing weight, but if you want to continue the diet for a long time, you need to look at other elements like whether you are getting enough dietary fiber and so on.

The Ikigai Diet is designed for a healthy individual to apply as a long-term eating habit, not to treat certain conditions.

## ARE ALL CARBS THE ENEMY?

According to Dr. Zenji Makita, who is the author of *Isha Ga Oshieru Shokujijutsu, A Diet A Doctor Recommends*, what you need to worry about is sugar, not necessarily carbohydrates. A carb can be problematic when it is broken down into sugar. He specializes in diabetes, and he has seen over 200,000 patients with diabetes.

He says there are some sugar rich foods you want to avoid more than others, and you need to understand the order of them before developing an obsession that all carbs are dangerous.

## A SCALE OF SUGAR RICH FOODS TO AVOID

1. Soft drinks such as coke. The first group to avoid is drinks that contain a lot of white sugar. Absorbing sugar in liquid state is the worst way, he says.

2. Sweets such as cakes and doughnuts. The second worst group is sweets containing a lot of white sugar.

3. Fruits. Fruits are better than the first two groups. And yet many of the fruit available today are engineered to have higher sugar content. Fruit juice is especially bad because it contains a lot more sugar than a fruit. When fruit juice producers make orange juice, for instance, they use 6 to 8 oranges, and you would end up ingesting more sugar than you would when you eat an orange.

4. White rice, white bread, noodles made from white flour such as pasta and ramen.

5. Brown rice, whole wheat bread, and potatoes.

He says that having white bread or white rice is okay, but you should reduce the amount. He doesn't say you shouldn't have them at all like some of the low carb diets suggest.

He also says that if you can, eat brown rice instead of white rice, and eat whole wheat bread instead of white bread. Yet, they too become sugar when they are broken down; therefore, you need to control the amount.

That is what Dr. Makita thinks. What about the position of the Ikigai Diet? What do I think we should do with white rice and brown rice? Before concluding, let's look at other research.

## CARBS IN SHORT-LIVED VILLAGES

Do you remember what the people in short-lived villages were eating?

White rice. They were eating a lot of white rice with salty pickles. Because they didn't have vegetable fields, they had to fill their stomach with rice, and to help eat rice, they ate some pickles with a lot of salt. They ate 4 to 7 bowls of rice with each meal. Among the short-lived villages, there were fishing villages, where they ate only rice and fish, no vegetables because they didn't have vegetable gardens, either.

It seems to suggest that eating a lot of white rice isn't good for us, and if you want to eat it, you can limit the amount to 1 or 2 bowls per meal.

The book *Long-lived Villages and Short-lived Villages in Japan* doesn't talk about brown rice. Perhaps, it is because most people in Japan don't and haven't eaten brown rice in the last 100 years or so. People have either eaten white rice or rice with other grains such as barley and millet. It is another misconception about Japanese people in the West that we eat brown rice. No, we don't. We ate brown rice up until the Edo period, which was about 200 years ago, but we started polishing rice from the Meiji era, and today most people eat white rice except Shizenha people. According to the book, people who ate white rice with other grains lived longer than people who ate only white rice.

It seems to suggest that it is also advisable to cook white rice with other grains such as barley and millet, if you want to eat white rice.

What about brown rice, then?

## THE THOUGHTS OF A NATURALIST DOCTOR

Another doctor Shinjiro Honma, the author of *Byoki Ni Naranai Kurashi Jiten, A Complete Guide to A Lifestyle without Getting Sick*, recommends brown rice because it has dietary fiber and detoxication mechanisms, which are helpful in today's diet, where we are often exposed to all kinds of chemicals.

Shinjiro Honma has a large following among Shizenha people because he has a holistic understanding of health both from his medical background and his natural lifestyle.

He graduated from Sapporo Medical University. Then he worked for the university hospital and Hokkaido Pediatric Center as a pediatrician. In 2001, he went to the National Institute of Health in the United States where he conducted research on virology and vaccinology for three years. After returning to Japan, he worked at the Neonatal Intensive Care Unit in Sapporo Medical University as the head of the unit. In 2009, he moved to Nasu-Karasuyama city in Tochigi Prefecture to begin leading a sustainable lifestyle while working at a local clinic called Nanago Clinic.

He grows vegetables using Natural Farming methods and makes fermented foods such as miso and soy sauce in the traditional way. With his knowledge of bacteria, which he gained from virology, he further researches them through his practice of farming and fermentation.

He is also familiar with oriental medicine, which helps him form a comprehensive understanding of health and medicine.

As a pediatrician, he often gives advice to people who practice natural parenting, especially in relation to bacteria and microbiota, how to deal with vaccination or germicides. He raises his children naturally, as well. He writes articles for a health magazine called *Sokai* and a natural parenting magazine called *Kuyon*. He gives talks throughout Japan on healthy eating, natural parenting, and how to deal with vaccination.

He says that watching your carbohydrate intake is okay if you want to do it, but you also need to think about your gut microbiota, and brown rice is one of the best foods for the gut bacteria. Like Zenji Makita, he suggests that you stop consuming sugar-filled foods such as soft drinks, sweets, and fruit juice first, then white rice and foods made of white flour, but you don't need to avoid eating brown rice.

He is not a big fan of bread, including whole wheat bread, because you need to bake it at very high temperatures, and he recommends to people that we should only eat bread occasionally. He is talking to the Japanese audience, by the way, whose diet didn't include bread originally. Our climate isn't suitable for growing wheat, so why do we go through all the trouble of harvesting it during the rainy season, and milling it, when we have a grain called rice? That's what he is saying. However, that isn't the case in many countries in the West. Therefore, it may not apply to you.

## BLUE ZONES- 30% OR 70% CARBS?

There is another element to consider. Do you remember Blue Zones? Five areas in the world where people lived the longest. Okinawa is one of them. People in Blue Zones have 50 to 80% carbs in their diets. Surprising, isn't it? Yet, the carbs they are eating are whole grains or the potato group such as sweet potatoes.

## BROWN RICE AND THE JAPANESE NATURAL FOOD MOVEMENT

Although brown rice hasn't been eaten among the members of the general public, it has been the staple food in the Japanese natural food movement. It was advocated by Sagen Ishizuka, who started the natural food group Shokuyokai at the beginning of the 20<sup>th</sup> century, and it has been part of the natural food culture since then.

## THE IKIGAI DIET ON CARBS AND BROWN RICE

Considering what Zenji Makita and Shinjiro Honma said, as well as the discovery of Shoji Kondo, and Blue Zones diets, what I think about carbs is that it is okay to eat brown rice.

We don't need to cut it down.

We should avoid white rice as much as possible, and if we want to eat it, have it with other grains such as barley or pearl barley.

We should avoid foods made from white flour as much as possible but can eat foods made from whole wheat flour such as whole wheat bread or whole wheat pasta, especially for the Westerners since they are very much part of your dietary culture.

I also recommend that you increase the frequency of eating oats and barley so you can diversify your grain consumption. It is also part of your dietary culture to have breakfast cereals, so having muesli and oatmeal with a lot of nuts and dried fruit is a good way of absorbing dietary fiber. I would choose organic ones without any added sugar and soak them in soymilk overnight. In this way, dried fruit will give sweetness.

Bread is okay as long as you eat whole wheat bread, sourdough bread, and bread with many other grains, but I still think you want to limit the amount. Instead, you can have wheatberries or oat berries, because they are closer to their original form, and match the concept of Ichibutsu Zentai Shoku, whole food. You don't need to mill them when you can eat them as they are, just like eating rice.

You can have potatoes, too, but not frying them. Steaming or boiling them is more advisable. You can also increase the frequency of eating sweet potatoes and taros.

# CHAPTER 7

# THE SUPERFOOD RICE ALTERNATIVES

# TO BROWN RICE

## ALTERNATIVES TO BROWN RICE

Brown rice is considered to be the most balanced food according to the macrobiotic diet, and it is popular worldwide. It is favored among Japanese naturalists, as well.

A lot of my friends eat it.

Recently, though, there are other alternatives among the health-conscious people in Japan.

### MUGIMESHI

Mugimeshi is one of them. It is white rice with barley or pearl barley. It is what many people ate in the long-lived villages. It was common throughout Japan since rice was a luxury. In other words, it was a peasant's meal, but ironically it turns out to be healthier because barley contains beta-glucan, which is soluble dietary fiber that is strongly linked to improving cholesterol levels and boosting heart health. It is catching the attention of many Shizenha people now.

### ZAKKOKUMAI

Zakkoku means miscellaneous grains or native grains such as barley, pearl barley, black rice, red rice, millet, buckwheat, and so on. Zakkokumai is a mixture of rice and Zakkoku. It was also a peasant's meal in the past, but it is becoming popular among Shizenha people now. Zakkoku is advocated a lot by a natural food diet called Miraishoku Tsubutsubu, which is one of the newer dietary practices I mentioned in Chapter 1. It is called Tubu-Tubu Future Food in English, and it has an English website. This is one example of how the Japanese natural food movement has evolved since the macrobiotic era. The practitioners of Tubu-Tubu Future Food often eat each type of native grains without mixing them with others, but other Shizenha people mix miscellaneous grains with rice and eat them as Zakkokumai.

Tubu-Tubu Future Food
http://tubu-tubu.net/

## HATSUGAGENMAI

Hatsugagenmai means sprouted brown rice. You soak brown rice for about two days, depending on the season, until the rice begins sprouting. By sprouting the rice, it increases GABA, gamma-Aminobutyric acid. It also makes the rice softer, and many people find it easier to chew than brown rice.

## KOSOGENMAI

Kosogenmai means fermented brown rice or enzyme brown rice. You soak brown rice with azuki beans and sea salt for about 12 hours, then you cook them in a pressure cooker. When they are cooked, you move them into a jar rice cooker and leave them there on the warm setting, about 70 degrees Celsius (158 Fahrenheit), and let them ferment for about three days. Make sure to mix the rice once a day to let oxygen in; it stimulates the fermentation process.

For details, please read the following blog post.
https://ikigaidiet.com/how-to-make-fermented-brown-rice/

By fermenting brown rice, it increases the nutrients tremendously, dietary fiber to 127%, protein to 115%, vitamin B2 to 125%, vitamin B1 to 134%, iron to 190%, calcium to 178% more. It is the ultimate superfood, having the benefits of whole food and fermented food. If you choose rice to be the staple food and to eat it every day, by absorbing it in its best state, it can have the most desirable effect on your diet.

I eat Kosogenmai every day, and sometimes, I put pearl barley berries in it to make it fermented brown Mugimeshi, or add other grains to make it fermented Zakkokumai.

If you can't get hold of azuki beans, black beans are also okay. You can make it without the beans, too, if you are not able to obtain any of them.

If you like, you can always sprout the rice before fermenting it, but I don't think that is necessary since regular fermented brown rice is already good enough. It takes a long time to make fermented sprouted brown rice.

# CHAPTER 8

## KYODO RYORI

## THE AUTHENTIC WASHOKU

## REGIONALITY OF KYODO RYORI

Kyodo Ryori means local cuisines in Japanese, and there are a whole variety of them in every region. When you say Washoku, you might think of sushi, tempura, or sukiyaki, or if you think of a more sophisticated version, you might picture Kaiseki Ryori, but they are just a small part of Japanese cuisines. When you travel in Japan, I highly recommend that you try the local cuisines of the area you are visiting because they are the authentic Washoku. They are healthier, too, since they usually use ingredients available in the region and the traditional cooking method suitable to the area, making them Shindofuji, local and seasonal.

For example, in Hino, Shiga, where I live, we have Hinona-Zuke, Koimo-No-Nikkorogashi, Tai-Somen, and many other dishes. Hinona-Zuke means Hinona pickles. Hinona is an heirloom radish grown in Hino, and Hinona-Zuke is our main pickle. Koimo-No-Nikkorogashi is stewed taros. Koimo is a type of taro potatoes similar to Satoimo, and we have an heirloom Koimo in Hino.

Tai-Somen means sea bream somen-noodles. It is a dish we eat on May 3rd when we have Hino Festival, the main festival in our town. We stew sea bream with various seasonings, and later we put somen-noodles in the soup and soak them until they absorb the sea bream flavor. The sea bream and somen we use are not necessarily local, so it is different from the former two dishes in that sense. Yet, it is considered to be a Kyodo Ryori since it is tied with our local culture.

## SLOW FOOD MOVEMENT

Have you ever heard of the Slow Food Movement? It is a movement led by an organization called Slow Food that promotes local food and traditional cooking. It began in Italy in 1986 and has since spread worldwide. As an alternative to fast food, it strives to preserve traditional and regional cuisines and encourages farming of plants, seeds, and livestock characteristic of the local ecosystem.

From Slow Food's point of view, eating Kyodo Ryori is Seken-Yoshi, socially friendly, by protecting the local farming and the local economy. It is also beneficial for your health from the viewpoint of Shindofuji.

In your region, too, there must be some local cuisines which have been passed down from generation to generation, and they are ingrained in your land and culture. They are the most suitable food in the climate of your area. The best thing for you is to find organic ingredients and cook them at home. You can also arrange the recipes a little to use ingredients that include Ma Go Wa Ya Sa Shi I or food filled with dietary fiber.

# CHAPTER 9

## WHEAT VS. RICE

## THE IKIGAI DIET FOR EUROPEANS

## SHINDOFUJI IN THE IKIGAI DIET

While many aspects of the Ikigai Diet are universal, such as natural food, fermented food, Ma Go Wa Ya Sa Shi I, Ichibutsu Zentai Shoku, and Ichiju Sansai, you need to take regional factors into consideration, from the viewpoint of Shindofuji.

## FINDING A COMPATIBLE BACTERIUM IS THE KEY

Brown rice is good for Europeans, too, since it has a well-balanced nutritional value, but it has a further benefit for East Asians who have been eating it as a staple food. According to Hitoshi Dozono, the inventor of a popular brown rice liquid called Bannokoboeki, brown rice bacterium is one of the two most powerful bacteria, along with the Natto germ, and it helps us Japanese keep the balance in the body. Therefore, we gain benefits not only from the nutrients but also from the germ. And it is because rice is our staple food, we have developed a strong bond with this bacterium.

What about Europeans, then?

You must have a bacterium that is compatible with your gene. Mr. Dozono thinks that it is usually in the staple food of the region.

In the case of Europe, wheat, oats, barley, rye, and potatoes are your staple foods. Historically, wheat has been eaten since ancient times, while potatoes came from South America in the 16th century, so I think the bacterium in wheat could be suitable to your genes.

## FERMENTED WHEAT BERRIES

I recommend fermented wheat berries as your way of absorbing wheat germ. You can make fermented wheat berries in the same way as making fermented brown rice. You soak wheat berries with azuki beans and sea salt for about 12 hours; then pressure cook them. When they are cooked, you move them into a jar rice cooker and leave them there on the warm setting, about 70 degrees Celsius (158 Fahrenheit), for three days. Make sure to mix the wheat once a day to let oxygen in; it stimulates the fermentation process. If you can't get a hold of azuki beans, black beans are also okay, or without the beans.

For details, please read the following blog post.
https://ikigaidiet.com/how-to-make-fermented-wheat-berries/

## FERMENTED SPELT BERRIES

Spelt seems to be even better since it is ancient wheat. You can try making fermented spelt berries. You can make them in the same way as fermented wheat berries.

## FERMENTED OAT GROATS

Oat is another option. You may want to experiment with different grains to see which one suits you, since it is a new concept. Many Japanese people have already eaten fermented brown rice and have experienced dramatic improvements in their well-being, but that is not the case in Europe. You may be used to eating oatmeal, but oats used for oatmeal are rolled oats. Oat groats are in their original form, and they are more aligned with the concept of Ichibutsu Zentai Shoku. You can make fermented oat groats in the same way as fermented wheat berries.

## FERMENTED BARLEY GROATS

The same thing can be said about barley groats. I have made all of them, actually; fermented wheat berries, fermented spelt berries, fermented oat groats, fermented barley groats, as well as fermented buckwheat groats. I have even mixed some of these grains with brown rice. You just need to try eating different grains to see which one suits you best.

You don't always have to ferment them. I have eaten all of them after pressure cooking them before putting them in a jar rice cooker, and they taste great as they are. It takes less time. Just like brown rice has nutritional value, they have the value of being a whole food. Fermenting them just adds benefits.

## FERMENTED ZAKKOKUMAI

If you want to avoid gluten, you can always have fermented Zakkokumai with brown rice, wild rice, buckwheat, quinoa, millet, and oats.

# CHAPTER 10

# THE SEVEN FOODS THAT WILL AGE YOU FASTER

## FROM A HEALTH POINT OF VIEW

I have been talking about what to eat so far. How about foods that we should avoid? If we get into the details, there are a lot of foods we are better off staying away from, for ethical reasons or environmental reasons, and so on, but here, I just want to focus on our health. Are they good for our body? Otherwise, the list goes on and on, and I don't want to let you pay attention to the foods we shouldn't eat that much. I will just give you a list of the worst of the worst.

## 1. SOFT DRINKS

Avoid soft drinks such as coke and soda. If you are reading this book, you probably don't drink any of those but just in case. As I wrote in Chapter 6, Dr. Zenji Makita says absorbing sugar in liquid state is the worst way.

## 2. SWEETS

Avoid sweets such as cakes, doughnuts, muffins, brownies, and chocolate bars as much as possible. If you want to eat something sweet, choose foods using raw sugar, honey, or natural syrups such as maple syrup instead of white sugar. And yet I think people in the West eat sweets way too much, including those considered more natural.

If there is one big difference between Japan and the West, I would say it's the amount of sugar intake, even if it is brown sugar. As I said before, in Japan, we don't have the custom of eating muffins or doughnuts for breakfast. For breakfast, we have rice, miso soup, a protein dish, and a vegetable dish. We don't have a custom of having sweets during our tea break. We drink green tea with pickles. We don't have the tradition of having dessert after dinner.

Unfortunately, this is changing now, a lot of young people have pastries for breakfast, and they often have cakes with their coffee at Starbucks for their afternoon breaks. In spite of that, we consume less sweets on the whole because it isn't our routine.

In the West, however, even among the health conscious people, you might have orange juice, granola, muffin, and coffee for breakfast. You might use brown sugar or honey as sweeteners, but when it adds up, it becomes a lot of sugar. Then you might have cakes or bread with jam for your coffee breaks. If you have dessert after dinner, the total amount of sugar intake will be a lot. You may be eating organic, vegetarian food, but it can be counterbalanced by all this sugar.

## 3. FRENCH FRIES, CHIPS, AND OTHER SNACKS

You want to avoid snacks in general, whether they are sweet or not, especially fried snacks like chips and French fries. Carbs which are fried with a high temperature around 120 degrees Celsius (248 Fahrenheit) are said to contain acrylamide, which is suspected of being carcinogenic.

## 4. PROCESSED FOOD

Stay away from processed foods as much as possible because they contain all kinds of additives. Think about it. If you mass produce food and sell it at supermarkets, you have to make sure that the food remains fresh for a long time, and to do it, you need to use artificial preservatives. It is always better to cook everything yourself.

It also means it is safer to eat at home than eating out, unless you find good natural food restaurants. In this way, you can choose the ingredients carefully, not only the main ingredients but also the type of oil and seasonings.

Some of the well-known processed foods are bacon and sausages. There is an interesting episode in Japan. A vegetarian person went to a restaurant and ordered a dish without meat. The waiter said "no problem" and brought a dish that had bacon in it.
"Excuse me, there is meat here," the customer complained.
"No, that's not meat, that's bacon."

It does happen a lot, actually. Although we were all vegetarians in the past, modern-day Japanese people don't know much about vegetarianism. They think you don't eat meat because you don't like it and maybe bacon is different. Well, from the health point of view, it is even worse than regular meat.

## 5. FRUIT JUICE

Even if it says 100%, fruit juice is usually made with a lot of fruit. For example, you might need between 13 and 15 oranges to produce a 1-liter bottle of orange juice (this changes depending on the size, of course). You absorb more sugar from drinking a glass of orange juice than eating an orange.

## 6. MEAT

I said meat was better than bacon, but still, it is one of the seven worst foods. I am sure you have heard of so many reasons to be a vegetarian, so I won't go into detail here. I can just add one more thing: It is more strenuous for your stomach and intestines to digest meat. Therefore, to protect your intestines, you are better off staying away from meat. We didn't eat meat in Japan for a long time. Meat came into our diet only about 150 years ago, and most people started eating meat on a regular basis in the 1960s when Japan entered the high economic growth period. That means many of the centenarians who are referred to as role models of longevity must have spent their childhood and early adulthood without eating meat.

Dr. David Sinclair, the author of *Lifespan: Why We Age—and Why We Don't Have To*, says that an excess amount of animal-based amino acids may accelerate aging, and he avoids eating meat, except chicken.

## 7. DAIRY PRODUCTS

Avoid milk and dairy products as much as possible. Dairy products weren't part of our diet until recently, either. Again, there are many websites giving reasons to stop consuming dairy products, so I won't go into detail here, but for one, a lot of the milk contains hormones and anti-biotics. Among the dairy products, cheese and yogurt are better because they are fermented. Both cheese and yogurt contain spermidine, an autophagy activating polyamine, and therefore they might help you live longer. For cheese, choose natural cheese, not processed, and for yogurt, choose plain ones without sugar.

## SLOWING DOWN THE ELEVATION OF YOUR BLOOD SUGAR LEVELS

What about carbs? Yes, there are some carbs you should avoid, too, but I don't want to make the list too long. As I have already indicated, I want to focus on foods that are good to eat, rather than thinking about foods we can't eat. I will talk about it more in detail later, but this is an important element of the Ikigai Diet; differentiating itself from other diets. These seven kinds of food are the essential ones that you want to keep in mind.

As I wrote in Chapter 6, you also want to avoid white rice, white bread, and foods made from white flour. Nevertheless, if it is too much to handle, there are ways to slow down the rising of your blood sugar level even if you eat them. Dr. Zenji Makita says that the order in which you eat your food can make a difference.

1. Vegetables
2. Protein such as meat, fish, and beans
3. Carbohydrate

So, if you have to eat white rice or white noodles, first eat some vegetables, and then beans or fish, before eating rice or noodles.

If you have olive oil or vinegar before or with carbs, it also slows down the rising of your blood sugar level. Therefore, if you eat bread or pasta, it is better to put olive oil on them.

I usually make a dressing with brown rice vinegar, olive oil or perilla oil, sesame seeds or hemp seeds, and sea salt. I put it on a salad and have it for the first thing in a meal. It is also good from the viewpoint of the raw food diet because you are absorbing enzymes more effectively by eating raw vegetables first.

# CHAPTER 11

## THE SECRET OF JAPANESE LONGEVITY

## HOW OVER WHAT

## SUMMARY SO FAR

Let me sum up what I have covered so far.

1. Use organically or naturally grown ingredients.

2. Use locally grown ingredients.

3. Eat and make fermented foods.

4. Eat whole food, Ma Go Wa Ya Sa Shi I, dietary fiber, and One Soup Three Dishes.

5. Not all carbs are bad for you; you don't need to avoid whole grains.

6. Eat fermented brown rice, wheat berries, oat groats, barley groats, and other grains.

7. Eat local cuisines.

8. Avoid consuming soft drinks, sweets, French fries, chips, other snacks, processed food, fruit juice, meat, and dairy products.

9. When you eat, eat vegetables first, then protein, and finally, carbs.

Now that you know what to eat and not to eat, in this chapter, I am going to discuss how to eat, since how you eat plays a significant role in our diet to stay healthy.

## ARE YOU EATING GREAT FOOD, BUT MAYBE A BIT TOO MUCH?

A lot of people in the West are conscious of what you eat, and I feel very positive about the way organic food culture is expanding. If there is one thing I feel lacking in the natural food movement in the West, however, is the way you eat. Generally speaking, people still tend to eat too much. In spite of the fact that you eat great food, if you put too much food in your stomach, the stomach cannot digest it well enough before passing it to the intestines, which will give the intestines more work to do.

## HARA HACHIBUNME

We have a saying called Hara Hachibunme, which means eating until 80% full. In other words, stop eating when your stomach is 80% full, not completely full. You feel a little hungry, and you could eat a bit more, but that is the time to put your fork down.

Always think of your stomach and intestines. Will it give them more work? Can they handle this amount of food?

## HOW MANY TIMES SHOULD YOU CHEW?

Chewing is another thing that can help your stomach digest food. It is the first stage of your digestion, and if you can break down food as much as possible in your mouth, it will be easier for the stomach to digest it, and it can pass the work to the intestines in a good state.

One reason why many people have damaged intestines is that they don't chew enough, which means their food isn't properly broken down as it goes into the pipes. This forces your bowels to work harder than they should as they try to break down the food.

So how many times should you chew?

According to the macrobiotic diet, to have healthy intestines, you ought to chew 100 times. However, I have heard a theory that chewing 25-30 times was enough for your guts. You just need to figure out for yourself which way is comfortable for you; comfortable for your stomach and intestines. It also depends on how much food you put in your mouth each time.

## SNACKING BETWEEN MEALS

You don't want to eat between meals either. This is because you want to give your digestive organs a break. If you have lunch around noon, and you have some cookies during your tea break around 3 o'clock, your stomach has only 2 and a half hours to rest. If you can wait until 6 o'clock to eat something, on the other hand, the stomach can rest for over 5 hours. If you want to eat your dessert, it is better to eat it with your lunch.

## INTERMITTENT FASTING

On the same note, you can skip a meal or meals to give your digestive system a break. In Japan, we used to have only two meals a day until around 1700 A.C. We didn't have breakfast and had lunch around noon and had dinner around 4 pm. It was very much like today's intermittent fasting, the one that you have 16 hours of not eating period each day. It is a good idea to bring back this tradition and have some hungry period.

Dr. David Sinclair, the author of *Lifespan: Why We Age – and Why We Don't Have To*, says that if you have a certain period of hunger, it can activate your longevity gene called sirtuin, and it will stop the aging process. Also, according to Dr. Atsushi Aoki, the author of *Kufuku Koso Saikyo No Kusuri, The Hunger is the Best Medicine*, intermittent fasting is one of the most effective ways to activate autophagy.

There are different methods of intermittent fasting, and you can do the one that suits your lifestyle. The 16/8 method is the most popular way in Japan, and I practice it, too. I finish eating dinner by 8 p.m. and don't eat until noon the next day. In other words, I skip breakfast. Because I include the sleeping time in the 16 hour fasting period, it isn't so hard. In my case, though, I do it five days a week, instead of the usual seven days a week practice. I have a logical reason for it, but I will explain it later.

From time to time, you can skip lunch, too, to give the digestive organs a longer break. You can do this once a week. You can also try one day fasting, skipping three meals, once a month.

## DRINKING WATER

It is good to drink a lot of water, too. It increases our saliva, and saliva aids in digestion. You can drink 1.5 liters-2 liters a day, depending on your body size. I always drink a glass of water the first thing in the morning since it cleanses our organs first.

# CHAPTER 12

## ADDING HYGGE TO THE JAPANESE DIET

## WHY THE HEALTH CONSCIOUS GET SICK

Do you know any people who practice things I have been recommending, and yet, for some reason, they often get sick?

If so, how could that be?

Well, one possibility is that these people were often sick before starting their diet and haven't regained their healthy condition yet. It is often the case that people who have health problems look into this kind of diet in the first place.

## PLACEBO EFFECT

Another possibility is the placebo effect. When we become health conscious, we tend to be more sensitive to what we eat. Let's say you decided to eat only organic vegetables, but you can't always eat organic vegetables because they are not available all the time. When you eat non-organic vegetables, you feel bad, and that makes you sick. However, if you don't care about what you eat, you can feel happy about anything you eat.

In Japan, we have a saying, A Fool Never Catches a Cold.

The mind is powerful. We do need to take our psychological aspects into consideration.

## ARE YOU TIRED OF PEOPLE TELLING YOU WHAT YOU CAN'T EAT?

One way that the Ikigai Diet is different from other dietary practices is that we don't set any rules on what you can eat and what you can't eat. It is all up to each person, and you can basically eat anything you like; even the seven kinds of food I suggested that you should avoid.

It is better to avoid them if you can, but it is also crucial that you find a way that is comfortable and doable for you. Every person is different, and you have your unique way that works for you. You don't have to follow exactly the same diet with others. Any diet can work for some people, whether it is the macrobiotic diet or raw food diet, or a low carb diet, but not for everybody. That applies to any other field, such as psychotherapeutic methods or learning methods. I know that from my experience of having tried many different approaches in various fields. The best way is to adjust the formula a little bit to make it suitable for you, instead of strictly following it. People who are successful with a diet tend to do that, including Japanese naturalists. Therefore in the Ikigai Diet, we give you that freedom to make it more effective for you.

## VEGETARIANS VS. LOCAL FOOD EATERS

You don't want to get hung up on one single issue, either. Some people make it a strong rule to be a vegetarian, for instance. If you ate meat, you committed a crime or something. While I understand and respect their point of view, I also know that by not eating meat at all itself doesn't solve the problem. In order to stop the meat production, the majority of the world population needs to stop consuming meat, not only a small percentage of the people, which is what is happening now. We need to get more people to stop eating meat or to eat less meat. Since we are all different, not everybody can follow a strict diet. If we make it easier, on the other hand, more people may be able to practice it, and it will reduce the overall meat consumption.

Whatever the conviction we have, it is only one part of a big picture. Other people may feel strongly about other things like local food, not using any plastic, not eating chocolate because it is causing child labor, not supporting fast fashion, or more. You might be a vegetarian but may be eating soybeans or almonds imported from another side of the planet. In that case, people who are convinced that global food culture is the source of evil might criticize you for not following their guidelines.

Who is righter? Vegetarians who eat imported food, or meat eaters who eat local food?

It depends on your conviction, isn't it? Each party can give us tons of facts to support their argument. The thing is, you can always find something if you look for them, and you also oversee things in the field you don't pay attention to. You know a lot about a field because you happen to be interested in it right now, but you don't know about all issues. And who knows, you might be feeling very strongly about something else in a few years.

So, instead of trying to prove that you are right, and criticizing others, we can respect one another for being a part of a bigger movement to transform society.

It would be best if you can pay attention to all issues and you can practice everything, but how many people do you know who live like that?

You can't do everything. You just need to try your best within your capacity.

It is better to be a vegetarian in many ways, but if you find it difficult to completely stop eating meat, you may want to apply this method instead.

Avoid eating animals close to you the most. It means animals with four legs. If you have to, it is better to eat chicken, and fish is even better because it is further away from us.

You also want to consider how meat is produced. Avoid eating meat that is produced through factory farming. If you want to eat meat, find meat that is produced in a more animal-friendly manner, such as grass-fed meat.

Or you can eat less. It is much better to eat meat once a week than every day. If you had been eating meat every day, by reducing it to once a week, you have reduced your meat consumption a great deal, and if stopping meat entirely was too much of a task, and this once a week policy was doable, having this option will make a lot of difference.

## HARE AND KE

We have a concept called Hare and Ke in Japan. Hare means not usual, and it is a time for festivals, celebrations, or ceremonies. Ke means usual, and it is our everyday life. We have feasts on days of Hare, but on other days that we call days of Ke, we eat simple dishes like rice, miso soup, and some pickles. In that sense, the one-soup-three-dish-meal is more for Hare. We dress differently and use different kinds of bowls and plates, as well on the days of Hare. By making a distinction between the two, we can appreciate the time of feasts more.

You can apply this custom to make a distinction between vegetarian days and meat-eating days. You can make your weekdays Ke and have simple vegetarian dishes and weekends be Hare and eat richer food, including meat.

In this way, you can appreciate meat a lot more, and your pleasure increases. On the other hand, if you eat meat every day, it becomes mundane, and you probably don't enjoy the taste that much. If that is the case, what is the point of eating meat? So it is a win-win for you: You are reducing your meat consumption while increasing the pleasure of eating.

The concept of Hare and Ke is the very reason I practice intermittent fasting five days a week and take a break on the weekend. Having the weekend off makes so much difference. Since intermittent fasting isn't for kids, my son has breakfast, and it is nice to be able to have breakfast with him on the weekend, where we often have our homemade pancake. I am refreshed on the weekend and get ready to start the regular routine on Monday, and on Friday morning, when I begin to feel the tension, I can say to myself, only four more hours to go. It is so much more doable. I call it Hare and Ke Intermittent Fasting and want to promote it.

## TRADITIONAL JAPANESE METHODS VS. MODERN JAPANESE METHODS

I am very much for enjoying life. The problem of traditional Japanese methods is that they can be rather serious, and everything becomes like a martial art training. You can probably be healthy and even enlightened by following them, but they aren't fun.

One of my missions in writing this book is to update the image of Japan, since many of the Japanese teachings introduced to the West have been brought by older generations, and they don't necessarily represent Japanese culture today. There is a reason why I chose young naturalists as our role models: Besides being the true successors of the traditional lifestyle; they carry a mentality that upgrades our culture.

The time when the older generations lived, we were not allowed to question the teacher; therefore, there was no room for improvement. In the last few decades, however, there have been a lot of changes made in Japan by younger generations challenging the authority. We have learned that only strictness will not help us reach enlightenment; neither will only relaxation. To take us to the next level, we need a good harmony between tension and enjoyment, and young naturalists have such balance.

## BRINGING HYGGE INTO THE JAPANESE DIET

The Ikigai Diet is like bringing a Danish element of hygge into the Japanese diet. After all, Danes are the role model for happiness. We can be a role model of longevity, but not happiness. Eating is hygge, and you want to be cozy and comfortable when you eat. On your day of Hare, you can put a beautiful tablecloth, light candles, and play enchanting music. Don't forget to have a good bottle of wine or sake as well.

## VEGETARIAN GOURMET FOODS

You don't need to always include meat in your feasts. Vegetarian dishes can be delicious, and you have a lot of hygge moments with them. Beans can replace meat in most recipes; you can make splendid pasta with soybeans, kidney beans, chickpeas, lentils, tofu, and Natto; you can make magnificent curry with most beans, and you can make mouth-watering dumplings with azuki beans. Again, you can find tons of recipes on the internet.

## ZEN AND THE ART OF MISO SOUP EATING

In my novel, *Miso Soup Romance*, the main character, Akira Takaoka, practices what he calls Zen and the Art of Miso Soup Eating. While he eats miso soup, he observes the vivid color of carrots and broccoli in the brown liquid; he smells the soup as he inhales the steam; then, he slowly picks the bowl and drinks the soup, feeling the liquid going down his gullet, releasing the neutral energy of fermented soybean curd to his entire organs, balancing Yin and Yang in them; finally, he begins chewing the vegetables, absorbing the dietary fiber in them. The whole act is a form of meditation for him. He also lights candles and plays classical music in the background.

Unfortunately, the novel is only available in Japanese, but you can practice Zen and the Art of Miso Soup Eating when you eat miso soup. You can do it with any dishes. Eating can be a form of meditation.

*Miso Soup Romance*
https://www.amazon.com/dp/B01JUW6MJG/

## SOCIALIZING ON A HEALTHY DIET

When you go on a particular diet, often you encounter moments when you can't follow your diet: For example, when you go to visit someone and served a meal not adherent to your diet. What do you do then?

I used to have this problem when I practiced the macrobiotic diet. At that time, I lived in England; I was a student at the British School of Shiatsu, where I studied macrobiotic Shiatsu. I could only hang out with macrobiotic people, and there were a limited number of them. It was one of the reasons why I stopped the diet. I switched to eating regular natural food since there were a lot more people whom I could share the diet with. I even extended my limit to regular Japanese food when I came back to Japan, since natural food culture was almost non-existent here, at least, among the general public.

Social life is vital for us, and sharing food is an essential element of it, and we do need to think of some measures to overcome this issue if we want to succeed in our diet.

Well, here is good news. I have heard that 70% of what you eat affects your health, not 100%. That's one of the reasons I am rather easy going about eating. It isn't the end of the world if you eat regular foods from time to time. You can relax a bit when you socialize with others. When served something you usually don't eat, you can think positively and appreciate the efforts of the person who cooked the meal, the farmers who produced the products, the sun, water, soil, and microorganisms that helped to produce the food. Spiritually speaking, that can change the vibration of the food. In other words, you can detoxicate the food by appreciating it.

As I noted earlier, the mind is powerful. How you feel affects your eating. While eating, you can visualize how the food is cleansing and energizing your body. Feel the nourishment spreading to all organs, bloodstreams, bones, muscles, and the brain.

## WHAT DO YOU DO WHEN YOU EAT OUT AND CAN'T FIND WHAT YOU CAN EAT?

It applies to when you eat out, too. I usually make exceptions when I eat out. We can try to find natural food restaurants or choose a healthier dish in a restaurant, but I prefer to forget about the whole thing and just have the food available there because quite often you have to exclude this and this to find a dish you can eat, and it isn't a complete meal. Sometimes, you end up complaining about the restaurant not having dishes you can have on their menu. If I have to feel negative, I might as well let it go and enjoy the dishes they have. Besides, it is fun to have something you usually don't have, and it is part of the reason you want to eat out in the first place.

## CREATE YOUR SOCIAL CIRCLE BY SHARING THE IKIGAI DIET

Having said that, it is better if you have a family and friends whom you can share your diet with. Then you can have weekly dinner parties with the Ikigai Diet. If possible, try introducing the Ikigai Diet to your family members and friends. The whole idea of the Ikigai Diet is Sanpo-Yoshi; you want to make it Aite-Yoshi, meaning make people close to you happy. Helping your family and friends lead a healthy lifestyle is critical so that you can protect them from lifestyle diseases. They, too, need a fit social circle they can share meals with, and you can support one another by being a positive influencer.

This is another reason I made the Ikigai Diet easy-going—so that many people can practice it. It is so much easier for you to introduce it to others than some of the stricter diets.

According to Dan Buettner, having a happy social circle is vital in Blue Zones, and it is one of their keys to longevity.

If you have families and friends who can influence one another positively and form a social circle that meets regularly to have birthday parties and weekly dinner gatherings, you are more likely to live long. You can even expand it to the entire community and transform your neighborhood into a Blue Zone.

To do this, you can start cooking for them. First, you can cook for your family based on the Ikigai Diet, and let them enjoy the food. Then you can begin inviting friends over to introduce the diet.

# CHAPTER 13

## IKIGAI DIET MENUS

## SUMMARY SO FAR

Now, let me sum up what I have covered in this book.

1. Use organically or naturally grown ingredients.

2. Use locally grown ingredients.

3. Eat and make fermented foods.

4. Eat whole food, Ma Go Wa Ya Sa Shi I, dietary fiber, and One Soup Three Dishes.

5. Not all carbs are bad for you; you don't need to avoid whole grains.

6. Eat fermented brown rice, wheat berries, oat groats, barley groats, and other grains.

7. Eat local cuisines.

8. Avoid consuming soft drinks, sweets, French fries, chips, other snacks, processed food, fruit juice, meat, and dairy products.

9. When you eat, eat vegetables first, then protein, and finally, carbs.

10. Stop eating when you are 80% full, chew a lot, and don't eat between meals or skip breakfast to give your gut plenty of breaks.

11. Drink a lot of water.

12. Don't become too strict about your diet and enjoy eating.

13. Use Hare and Ke to balance your diet.

14. Bring hygge and Zen into your dinner and make your eating a cozy and sacred experience.

15. Make exceptions when you socialize with others or eat out.

16. Create a social circle that can influence one another positively.

Now you have an overview of the Ikigai Diet; you can start applying it in your daily diet. The idea is balance and diversity. You want to include Ma Go Wa Ya Sa Shi I plus grains as much as possible in your daily meals. They can give you the nutritional balance; vitamins, minerals, protein, fat, and carbs. They also provide you with a wide variety of fiber to feed your gut microbiome. You don't have to have all of them in each meal, but try to design your meals so that you can consume them each day.

You also want to think about the omega-6 to omega-3 ratio. A healthy ratio of omega-6 to omega-3 fatty acids is said to be between 1.5 to 1 and 3 to 1. Generally, you consume way too much omega-6 fatty acids, so try to increase omega-3 intake by including blue-skinned fish in your diet or using omega-3 oil such as perilla oil and linseed oil in your dressings.

For fish, though, you don't want to have it every day, if you are over age 30, maybe just a few times a week, because the amount of amino acids called methionine, isoleucine, leucine, valine, and arginine is high, which can activate mTOR, and Dr. David Sinclair says it is preferable to suppress mTOR for anti-aging. To reduce the intake of these amino acids, you are better off staying on a plant based diet as much as possible.

In this chapter, I would like to give examples of what you can have for each meal.

## BREAKFAST

If you want to practice the 16-hour fast, you can skip breakfast. In my case, I have a glass of water the first thing in the morning, and then after doing my morning exercises, which I will explain later, I have a cup of organic black coffee, which helps me cope with fasting. I might have another cup of coffee, but I usually switch to drinking green tea for the second cup because green tea has a polyphenol called catechin, and catechin helps activate autophagy, according to Dr. Tamotsu Yoshimori, the author of *Life Science*.

For people under age 30, I don't think intermittent fasting is necessarily helpful. You may want to have breakfast. In that case, fermented brown rice with nori, miso soup, and a protein dish would be one breakfast option. You can put a lot of vegetables in the miso soup. In this way, you get enough veggies, and you don't need to make another vegetable dish. You use konbu as broth in the soup and put wakame, as well. For protein, you can have Natto or an egg dish provided that you use free-range eggs.

You don't have to eat a Japanese way; you have a great breakfast called muesli. A bowl of muesli contains a lot of dietary fiber from several grains, nuts, seeds, and dried fruit. You can have it with soy milk or soy yogurt, and it becomes a perfect breakfast. When you choose soy milk, make sure you get the kind made with organic and GMO-free soybeans. You can soak muesli in soy milk overnight so that the grains become soft and easy to digest. Soaked dried fruit gives sweetness, and you don't need to add sweeteners.

You can make a muesli bowl with fermented whole grains, meaning fermented brown rice, wheat berries, oat groats, and barley groats. Then you add nuts, seeds, and dried fruit.

Bread is another option. I don't recommend that you eat bread every day, but a few days a week would be okay. If you love bread, you want to have a hygge moment with it. I love bread with coffee in the morning, too. So I sometimes have bread for breakfast on the weekend, Hare period. It makes me feel good, and it is important to have such a happy feeling when you eat. You just need to make sure that you limit it to a few days a week and have muesli or fermented whole grains for the rest of the week.

I usually make bread myself. I mix whole wheat flour, rice flour, muesli, and fermented brown rice to make my original bread. Being able to choose the ingredients is one of the advantages of making your own bread.

I have a slice with olive oil or tahini. As I said before, olive oil slows down the rising of your blood sugar level, and therefore it is good to have with your bread or pasta. I usually have bread with salad and omelet, as well to make it more nutritionally well balanced. I sometimes steam bread instead of toasting it because bread is already dry after being baked. Toasting will make it even more dehydrated.

## LUNCH

For people practicing the 16 hour-fast, you want to make sure that you get enough nutrition from lunch and dinner. You want to think about the nutritional balance. Lunch is the first meal to break the fast; therefore, you want to eat a vegetable salad first to avoid a blood sugar spike because your blood sugar level is very low after 16 hours of fasting. Next, you have a protein dish and, finally, carbs. You don't need to finish the salad and protein dish before having carbs but eat a little bit of them first.

Let's say you are eating lunch at home. You can make it One Soup Three Dishes or One Soup Two Dishes.

Carbs: A bowl of fermented whole grains of some sort.
Soup: Miso soup with seaweed, seasonal vegetables, and tofu.
Pickles: Pickled seasonal vegetables
Dish 1: A pressure steamed small fish such as mackerel.
Dish 2: A salad with seasonal veggies and seeds or nuts with a dressing made of brown rice vinegar, sea salt, and olive oil or perilla oil.
Dish 3: Stewed or steamed root vegetables

When you pressure steam mackerel for about 30 minutes, borns will be soft enough to eat, and you can eat the whole thing. If you are eating sardine, you don't have to pressure steam it; just steaming it for 10minutes will make the borns soft enough. For dish 1, you can have any kind of protein dish, steamed soybeans, kidney beans, or chickpeas. Instead of putting tofu in your miso soup, you can make a tofu dish here, too.

For dish 2 or dish 3, you can have steamed, or stirfry vegetables, too. For ways of cooking, boiling, steaming, and stewing are better than stirfrying, and you want to avoid deep frying as much as possible. Fried foods can increase Rubicon, a negative regulator of autophagy, according to Dr. Tamotsu Yoshimori.

For oil, it is better to use omega-3 oil like perilla oil or omega-9 oil like olive oil instead of omega-6 oil. Because you can't heat up omega 3 oil, it is better to use it in a dressing, and you can put the dressing not only on a salad but also on a steamed vegetable dish.

Another way of using vinegar other than in a dressing is to make Sunomono, vinegared vegetables. The most common one is vinegared cucumbers and wakame seaweed. You put sliced cucumbers and wakame in a bowl with brown rice vinegar and soy sauce for about 30 minutes. It is another way of eating seaweed, too. You want to eat as many different kinds of veggies as you can, so it is good to have several dishes.

## SANDWICHES FOR LUNCH?

If you have lunch in your office, you can make a lunch box. You can make similar dishes for the lunch box, except the soup. You just have to give up the soup in this case.

Sandwiches are the most common form of a lunch box in the West. You can make sandwiches with whole wheat bread, too, but the problem with sandwiches is the portion of carbohydrate is way too high. Unless you put a lot of lettuce and tomatoes, you can't get enough vegetables. I think it is better if you make a lunch box with fermented whole grains with 2 to 3 side dishes.

## DINNER

For dinner, you can have One Soup Three Dishes or Two Dishes like lunch.

Carbs: Sweet potatoes or Taros. If you had grains for lunch, you can have potatoes for dinner to cover I of Ma Go Wa Ya Sa Shi I, but you don't have to do that every day. A few times a week is enough. You can have potatoes for lunch and grains for dinner, too. Remember, sweet potatoes are the staple food of Okinawans.

Soup: Miso soup with seaweed, seasonal vegetables, and tofu.

Pickles: Pickled seasonal vegetables

Dish 1: Natto. Natto is the most powerful superfood, in my opinion, and I recommend that you have it at least once a day. Although you can have Natto for any meal, the best time to have it is at nighttime because an enzyme called nattokinase in Natto, which is said to help you make your blood flow smoothly, works for 10 to 12 hours and it is good for it to work during your sleep.

Dish 2: Boiled or steamed leafy vegetables with sesame seeds or nuts

Dish 3: Steamed or stewed root vegetables. The idea is diversifying vegetables, whether they are root or leafy.

## SAY GOODBYE DESSERTS

Having sugar at night isn't recommended—no dessert after dinner. One big difference between Japan and European culture is having a custom to have dessert at night. Ice cream is one of the most common desserts isn't it? It is one of the worst foods you can have, and having it at night is the worst timing to have it because you usually don't move after dinner. If you want a dessert, have it after lunch. This way, you move after absorbing sugar, and moving can reduce the rising of your blood sugar level.

## THE PROS & CONS OF ALCOHOL

If you want to drink something, you can drink one or two glasses of wine. It is also a custom for Sardinia, Italy, and Icaria, Greece, in the Blue Zones. It is one of their nine factors of longevity.

According to Dr. Zenji Makita, grape wine and hard liquor like whiskey and shochu don't have much sugar compared to beer or rice wine. Therefore, he thinks it is better to drink wine or shochu. From observing his patients, he feels they are in better condition when they drink these kinds of alcohol than not drinking at all, provided that they don't drink excessively. It seems to suggest that a moderate amount of alcohol is actually better for our health.

Shochu is popular Japanese alcohol, and in Okinawa, people drink shochu called Awamori, regularly, and this could be another cause of their long life.

I think it has a psychological element, as well. Alcohol puts us in a better mood, and it helps us release our stress.

Drinking alcohol is very much part of our dining culture, so why not embrace it without damaging our health?

Selecting the right kind of alcohol is one way.

Controlling the amount is another way. With the same concept as Hara Hachibunme, stopping eating when we are 80%full, we can stop drinking when we are half drunk. Instead of getting drunk, we can enjoy the taste of wine, and feel the sensation of getting tipsy. Usually, the first few glasses are the most fun part, aren't they? Then, why not stop there?

We can always drink slowly to savor the moment longer. In other words, don't depend 100% on alcohol to give you a buzz—experience the moment through all of your senses, the color of the food, the smell, the music in the background, and the quality of your conversation. You can have uplifting conversations to feel high. That is much more exhilarating than the buzz you get just from drinking.

Well, I know it is hard to stop when you are getting into the mood of drinking. Then switch to tea. Herb tea or green tea would be good alternatives. Drinking water in between is also good. I usually stop drinking after two glasses of red wine, but if I want a third glass, I make sure to drink a glass of water before that. I always drink a glass of water before going to bed when I drink alcohol.

From time to time, you can drink until you are wasted, to let yourself completely go, but limit it to once or twice a month.

One of the reasons I take a break from intermittent fasting on the weekend is that I want to enjoy drinking. During the week, I only drink once every two days, and I have up to two glasses of wine and finish drinking by 8 pm, the same time as dinner. This is because wine does have calories, and you want to restrict your calorie intake completely during your fasting period. The only beverages you can drink are water, green tea, black coffee, or black tea. However, from time to time, I want to drink 3 or 4 glasses until late, and this system works perfectly. You can make the same exception for food and have meat and dairy on the weekend.

## PLAN A WEEKLY MENU

The idea is to cover Ma Go Wa Ya Sa Shi I plus grains as much as possible each day, but you can't always cover everything in a day. In that case, you can try to cover them each week. For example, if you ate only grains for carbs yesterday, you can have potatoes today, and so on.

Plan your meals for the entire week so that you can keep a good balance of Ma Go Wa Ya Sa Shi I, plus grains.

# CHAPTER 14

# IKIGAI EXERCISES

## THE IKIGAI DIET LIFE

The Ikigai Diet isn't just a diet; it is a lifestyle since everything else is related to our way of eating and wellness. What you eat and how you eat is probably the most important measure toward your well-being, and by changing your diet, you have increased your health and longevity. Nonetheless, it is always better to work on other areas, too, and Shizenha people lead a holistic lifestyle, eating well, exercising regularly, living in a natural environment, and working on their mentality. If you want to model them, you want to model all aspects of their life.

They, too, have similar factors to the ones elderlies in Ogimi village in Okinawa have.

1. They keep a vegetable garden

2. They belong to some form of a neighborhood association

3. They celebrate all the time with music and dance

4. They have an Ikigai, an important purpose in their life

5. They are proud of their tradition and local culture

6. They are passionate about everything they do

7. They help each other

8. They are always busy doing something

For the second factor, Belonging to a Neighborhood Association, they don't always belong to their local neighborhood association, but often they have a network of friends who lead a sustainable lifestyle locally. They have a support system similar to the local one, but it is often better because the way they communicate with one another is a new way, respecting the members' freedom and individuality. Sometimes, traditional neighborhood associations can be stressful due to their conforming nature. You are always worried about the eyes of your neighbors. You need to keep your yard weedless, for example.

For the third element, Celebrating All the Time with Music and Dance, it isn't common among the country elderlies in the main island of Japan, but young naturalists embrace arts such as music and dance a lot more, making them closer to Okinawans.

You sometimes see them bringing a djembe to the rice field and playing it while working there.

For the fourth part, Having an Ikigai, they have a clearer Ikigai than elders in general since they moved to the countryside with a purpose. They chose this lifestyle, and they have a mission to change the world by living sustainably.

For the fifth factor, Being Proud of Their Tradition and Local Culture, they are prouder of tradition and local culture since they are here to restore it.

For the sixth element, Being Passionate About Everything They Do, they are more passionate because they are young and have visions for their future.

For the eighth factor, Always Busy Doing Something, they move a lot like local elderlies working in the vegetable fields and rice fields. On top of that, they go cycling, walking, and mountain hiking.

From this chapter, I would like to share with you things you can do for your health and longevity other than eating.

First, let me cover exercises.

Any form of exercise is good for your well-being, whether it is a ball sport, working out at a gym, doing yoga, or outdoor activity. Therefore, do whatever you like doing. Depending on your age, too, different types of exercises are effective. Here I will introduce some exercises that can be done easily among the middle-aged and older since you are the ones who are more concerned about health. These are also easily done in the countryside, and they have other benefits than just being workouts.

### GARDENING

Many of the young naturalists grow vegetables, and some of them grow rice. Gardening is common among the people in Blue Zones, too, and this is part of their daily exercises. It is simply good as an exercise, but it has further benefits. You are constantly in touch with microorganisms in the soil, which enhance your immune system as gut microbiota does. You also become aware of the natural rhythm by working according to the weather and season, observing how plants grow and how insects live.

### WALKING

Walking is another common activity seen in many parts of the Blue Zones. It is better than jogging since you don't damage your knees, plus it is less strenuous to practice it daily. Walking is good for your mind, too, since you can relax while you are walking. When you jog, on the other hand, you feel a little tense. You can experience a state called runner's high after running for a while, but until you get to that state, you go through a painful period, and you might end up stopping before getting high. When you walk, you feel comfortable from the beginning, and after walking briskly for thirty minutes or so, the brain starts producing beta-endorphin, and you feel high. Having a relaxed mentality is crucial for a stress-free life.

### MOUNTAIN HIKING

Japanese people hike mountains a lot because about 70% of our land is covered by mountains, there are mountains everywhere, and mountain hiking is one of the most popular recreational activities in Japan. In the past, and still true in many rural parts of Japan, people hike mountains for religious rituals. Every village has a Shinto shrine, and a nearby mountain is often an object of worship. Many shrines are located on top of a mountain or halfway up a mountain, and people have to walk up the stone steps to get there.

I think our custom of hiking mountains is one of the causes of our longevity. I said that walking was a common daily activity in the Blue Zones, and it is walking up and down the hills in many parts. Therefore, it is more like mountain hiking. It isn't surprising that Nagano Prefecture has had the second-highest life expectancy in Japan in recent years since it is one of the most mountainous regions in Japan. When I lived in Nagano in my teens, I walked about eight kilometers (five miles) roundtrip to go to school. My house was located at 800 meters (2625 feet) above sea level, and the school was located at 600 meters (1969 feet) above sea level, which meant I walked down 200 meters (656 feet) on the way and walked up 200 meters on the way back. It was just like mountain hiking every day.

It is a lot harder than regular walking. In that sense, it is closer to jogging. As a physical work out, it is effective. However, as a mental exercise, walking on a flat land gives us more relaxation. On the other hand, mountain hiking provides us with another benefit, that is the connection with nature. It has the same effect as Shinrinyoku, forest bathing. We absorb Ki energy from the trees, and listening to birds soothes our mind.

If you don't have mountains in your region, you can always go walking on flat land, and hiking on a hill is also okay.

## NORDIC WALKING

What I recommend the most, if you live in plain fields, is Nordic walking. It is a sport from Finland, walking with two poles. The great thing about it is that your spine gets straight while walking. Kosuke Hirai, an acupuncturist who specializes in adjusting people's postures, says that our posture is the most important factor for our health. He is also a master of an ancient Japanese martial art, which was passed down from generation to generation in his family, and keeping the right posture in your daily movement is considered to be critical in his martial art. Having a straight back while walking is one of them, and how you walk determines your physical condition since it is something we do all the time. Nevertheless, most of us don't have a straight back when we walk, and the more we walk, the more we are actually damaging ourselves. Therefore, he thinks we should correct our posture before walking, and if we walk with two poles, our spine naturally becomes straight.

I started going Nordic walking after hearing about it from Mr. Hirai and found that it is true. The poles do make your back straight, and after going Nordic walking many times, you condition yourself to have your spine straight even without poles. In other words, Nordic walking is good training for you to walk with your back straight.

It has the same effects as regular walking, but Nordic walking has the benefit of correcting your posture.

I came up with something else that can further power-up Nordic walking, but I will introduce it to you in later chapters when I talk about mental work.

## HIIT

High-intensity interval training is becoming popular in Japan as an exercise to activate autophagy. I do it after Nordic walking three times a week during my intermittent fasting. I do push-ups, sit-ups, and squats as my HIIT so that I can also train my muscles. Muscle training is important when you do intermittent fasting because you might lose your muscles a little by fasting, and combining it with muscle workouts, intermittent fasting becomes more effective. As you get old, your muscles get weaker, and that can cause some injuries. By doing both Nordic walking and high-intensity interval strength training, it becomes a holistic workout combining aerobic and muscle exercises.

I do it, but HIIT can be a little too strenuous for people over 60, and you don't have to do it if you feel it is too hard. Going Nordic walking or walking is enough. Nobody in Blue Zones does HIIT, after all. Instead, you can emulate their habit I will share with you next.

### MOVE NATURALLY

People in Blue Zones and Japanese countrysides are constantly on the move, doing some kind of house chore. Gardening is one of them, and also, many other things like fixing things, chopping firewood, and making fermented food. They don't go to the gym or go running, but through their daily living, they get enough workouts. If you don't have time to do exercises, you can always incorporate them into your routine. Use stairs instead of the elevator, and use a bike instead of the car. Or walk when you have to go to the post office and other stores. Walking within the house can be an exercise if you move one room to another many times. When you finish eating, get up and take the dishes back to the kitchen and do the washing up right away. Dr. Zenji Makita says, moving right after eating slows down the rising of your blood sugar level, too, and it is good to do something. Lying on the sofa or taking a nap is the worst thing to do after eating.

## OUTDOOR SPORTS

Shizenha people enjoy outdoor sports. Engaging in outdoor activities is one of the perks of living in the countryside. Canoeing, mountain biking, or snowboarding are good ways to combine exercise and spending time in nature. I have a mountain bike, too. I don't cycle on a mountain trail since I am a little too old for that, but I cycle on flat off-road. It is quite fun and doable for middle-aged people. Cycling, in general, is good. I do what I call Satoyama cycling, which is to cycle in the countryside. I ride my bike along rice paddies to the library or for grocery shopping. It is a routine, but I get to enjoy the view at the same time.

## TRAIN YOUR INTERNAL ORGANS

Eastern exercises like Yoga, Taichi, and Qigong are wonderful ways to support your well-being. They are based on a holistic understanding of your health, and therefore more compatible with the Ikigai Diet. They, too, work on your gut and other organs in your body. Having Shiatsu or acupuncture treatments regularly is another option because they work on your energy lines called meridians, which are connected to your organs.

Training your muscles is a thing of the past; training your internal organs will be a new trend from now on.

## BODYWEIGHT TRAINING AND STRETCHING

If you want to do resistance training, it is better to do a bodyweight exercise like push-ups than lifting a barbel because you don't want to tense up your muscles so much, you want to soften them, as well. It is best done combining with stretching. A lot of us have the idea that it is better to have big muscles, but in oriental perspective, muscles need to be flexible as well as being strong.

# CHAPTER 15

## IKIGAI MINDSET

## THOUGHTS CAN AFFECT YOUR GUT

In Chapter 12, Adding Hygge to the Japanese Diet, I talked about how your mind affected your health. Recent studies show that your gut is related to your brain and how you eat influences your brain function. Therefore, eating gut-friendly food may be able to help diseases like dementia or autism. The researchers of these studies think it works the other way round, meaning how you think affects your gut and therefore influences your physical condition.

There are other studies suggesting that high subjective well-being (such as life satisfaction, absence of negative emotions, optimism, and positive emotions) causes better health and longevity.

Having a positive mentality when you eat is crucial, and that is the reason we don't set rules in the Ikigai Diet. When you set rules of what you can eat and can't eat, often, you feel negative when you face a situation where you encounter foods you can't eat.

In Chapter 10, The Seven Foods That Will Age You Faster, I said that I didn't want to make the list of bad foods too long because I wanted to focus on foods that are healthier to eat, rather than thinking about foods we can't eat. What you pay attention to is important. Even though you are eating the same kinds of food, choosing the foods because they are good, or choosing the foods by avoiding all harmful ones makes your mindset different.

In the Ikigai Diet, we are introducing a lot of wonderful foods and ways of eating, such as fermented foods, Ma Go Wa Ya Sa Shi I, Nimono, Sunomono, Aemono, Ichibutsu Zentai Shoku, Shindofuji, and one soup three dishes. Because they are so fabulous, we want to eat them all the time, and as a result, there is no room left for the seven worst foods.

Yes, there are times you might end up eating some of them. If this happens, what the heck? You might as well enjoy it. Always stay positive, no matter what. Your mind is sending signals to your body all the time, and you want to feed yourself with healthy thoughts just like you are choosing what to eat.

In other words, thoughts are foods, too. A diet should include your mentality.

## HOW TO STAY POSITIVE

You want to stay positive even when you are not eating. If thought is food, every time you think of something, you are feeding yourself. You want to practice positive thinking. It is often practiced for your happiness or success, but it is effective for your health, as well.

You want to live every day as if you are a healthy person. One method of modeling is that you model the mindset of your role model. Feel as if you are the role model. You have a healthy gut microbiota, and your organs are working fine.

You want to condition yourself to look at the positive aspects of your life. One way is to pay attention to your past successful experiences. Try to remember things that once had been your dreams but had become realities. For example, you wanted to learn a new language and you have mastered it, or you wanted to buy a house and you have bought one, or you wanted to start a business and you have started it. We tend to forget about those accomplishments once we achieve them. Instead, we think about things we haven't obtained yet, and feel inadequate. We wish we could speak another language, we wish we lived in a bigger house, or we wish the business we started had more sales, and so on.

It is a foolish way of using our brains. It is good to have new goals and strive toward them, but we don't want to stop enjoying our past successful experiences. Otherwise, it would be an endless game, and we would never be satisfied. Even if we make our new dreams come true, we will be feeling exactly the same as now.

You can list all your past successful experiences, and cherish them. I call it past successful experience meditation, and do it daily. It increases your self-esteem. You will feel you are successful, and it will make you feel happy and positive all the time.

## NO PAST SUCCESSFUL EXPERIENCES?

What if you don't have any successful experiences in the past? Most of us have some experiences of manifesting realities that once had been our dreams.

How many of us are living in neighborhoods we once dreamed of living in? How many of us dreamed of having a life partner and now have one? How many of us are in a field of work we always wanted to work in? How many of us are now in shape after working out for some time? How many of us desired to drive a car when we were a teenager and now drive one?

We should take advantage of small victories such as the ones stated above. Unfortunately, many of us don't see them as successes. We say things like, "So what if I'm married? Everyone is. I can't call that a success." When we hear that driving a car is a success, we say things like, "I drive a Honda Civic; success is driving a BMW." However, the main question is, wasn't there a time we didn't have all these things, and we desperately needed them?

## SHINON KANSHA: THE SECRET JAPANESE WAY OF PRAYING

There is something similar to past successful experience meditation. It is called Shinon Kansha. It means to appreciate the graces of the gods. This is the authentic way of praying at a Shinto shrine. Many people go to a shrine and ask for graces, but truly spiritual people don't do that. A shrine is a place where you give thanks to the gods for the favors they have already given to us.

I always appreciate the gods for manifesting my past accomplishments when I go to a shrine. I also acknowledge all of the great things happening in my life. They may not necessarily be my successful experiences, but they are things I can feel grateful for: The fact that I live in the countryside; the fact that I have a lovely family; the fact that I have time to go Nordic walking; the fact that I have a garden to grow vegetables, and so on.

I try to pay attention to those positive aspects of my life whenever I can. I try to occupy my thought with them. Of course, there are things I am not so grateful for happening in my life, too, but I don't have to pay attention to them. If I am busy thinking about happy things, I don't have time to notice the negative aspects of my life.

It helps with relationships, too. We do get annoyed by people around us at times, and yet we can always look at the bright side of them. Every person has a quality that provides us positive outcomes, no matter how irritating he or she can be in other areas. Then pay attention to that quality and enjoy the opportunity the gods have given to us.

## SHINON KANSHA NORDIC WALKING

I sometimes do Shinon Kansha during Nordic walking. I said that you could meditate while you walk, and this is especially good when you go Nordic walking because your spine is straight. In Zen meditation, the key is to have your spine straight, and the same thing can be said in walking meditation. When you walk with your back straight, you connect the heaven and earth, and you are more in tune with the universe. You can meditate in any way you like. You can just pay attention to what you see, the sounds, the smells, and the physical sensations. Or you can listen to your breathing. You can even recite a mantra. I like to do Shinon Kansha as my meditation. I list all of the things I feel grateful for and appreciate the gods for manifesting those realities. If you don't like to use the word gods, you can appreciate nature, the universe, or yourself for manifesting the outcomes.

## STRESS-FREE MENTALITY

One thing centenarians have in common is that they have a stress free lifestyle. They all have ways to shed stress, but many of them don't feel stressed in the first place because of their positive outlook on life. I am not a centenarian yet, but I am confident that I will be one because this is exactly the kind of mindset I have. I don't worry about things. I am easygoing and don't hold on to things. If something negative happens, I let it go and move on. Whatever happens in your life, it always leads to something else, and even it seems to be a crisis in the beginning, it can turn to an opportunity.

# CHAPTER 16

## SATOYAMA LIVING

## WHAT IS SATOYAMA?

Many of Shizenha people, Japanese naturalists, live in the countryside and lead what I call the Satoyama Lifestyle.

In Japanese, the word Satoyama symbolizes sustainability. Sato means livable or arable land, and the word Yama means mountains or hills. The word Satoyama usually describes an area that has mountains, forests, residences, and rice or vegetable fields. The reason why Satoyama stood for sustainability was its ability to self-sustain by circulating resources within an area.

What normally happens in a Satoyama is that the mountains that are sources of rivers supply water to the rice fields, and to the residents. The village then uses the trees on the mountains to build houses and furniture. The cutting down of trees also helps the forest survive because the spaces created will give way to sunlight that the young trees need to grow.

The remaining wood from the trees is collected together with the fallen leaves where humans then use the wood as firewood and the fallen leaves as fertilizers for their rice fields. After the people harvest the rice from the rice field, they end up with rice bran that they can use as fertilizers.

As you can see, the ecosystem was highly sustainable since each party was beneficial to the other. The Japanese people used to practice the Satoyama economy, a localized economy where everyone depended on the circulation of resources. These people farmed locally and grew diverse foods because that was what sustained the ecosystem.

Shizenha people try to live in Satoyama by circulating the resources within. Dr. Shinjiro Honma, the naturalist doctor I mentioned earlier, says that the key to maintaining your health is living in tune with nature. By growing your own food, you come in contact with microorganisms in the soil. By making your own fermented food, you release good bacteria into the house. By rising early in the morning and going to bed early at night, you live in tune with the natural rhythm.

This is the lifestyle common to people in Okinawa, Nagano, and Shiga.

If you can, move to the countryside and lead a Satoyama lifestyle. In many ways, it is so much easier to practice the Ikigai Diet in the countryside.

## SEASONAL WILD HERBS

One advantage of living in the countryside is that you can find edible wild herbs easily. Wild herbs are truly Shindofuji, local and seasonal. They contain local bacteria and can be found only at the right season. You won't be eating summer wild herbs in the spring, unlike imported fruit or greenhouse vegetables.

## COOKING ON WILDFIRE

Another benefit of country living is that you can cook on wildfire more easily. Some old houses have traditional style stoves where you use firewood for cooking. If you don't have one, you can always have a barbecue or Dutch oven cooking in your garden. The energy you get is different if you cook over natural fire, so I recommend that you do it from time to time. By the way, if you have an electric cooker, it is better to use a gas cooker, let alone a microwave oven.

## LIVING WITH CELESTIAL RHYTHM

When you live in the countryside, you can enjoy star gazing at night, and that makes you more aware of the stars and the moon. You can celebrate every new moon and full moon, or equinoxes and solstices. You can live in accordance with the celestial rhythm.

Conducting a ceremony at every new moon and full moon is especially good so that you can live with the lunar cycle rather than the monthly cycle in the Gregorian calendar. It was the way ancient people lived, and we had used the lunar calendar until the Edo period in Japan, too. Even today, some farmers use the lunar calendar to decide when to plant. It is more in tune with the natural rhythm.

By practicing a Satoyama lifestyle, you are more likely to live with your Ikigai and lead a happy life. I will explain more in the next chapter, which will be the final chapter.

# CHAPTER 17

## HOW TO FIND AND LIVE YOUR IKIGAI

## Ikigai and the Okinawan Myth

The Ikigai Diet is a diet to help you lead a long and healthy life. It is a diet to help you stay young until your final moments, but most importantly, it is a diet to lead a happy life. To be truly happy, you need an Ikigai.

Dan Buettner says that Ikigai is one of nine factors that contribute to the longevity of the people in Blue Zones. The word became well-known as an Okinawan concept, but it is used throughout Japan. It is a Japanese word. Just like the plant-based diet and the rural lifestyle of Okinawans are typical diet and lifestyle in most Japanese country villages, the concept of Ikigai isn't unique to Okinawans.

## Ikigai is not a Venn Diagram

So what does Ikigai mean? Ikigai means something that is worth living, rewarding, or fulfilling. You can find Ikigai in almost anything as long as you feel joy and meaning in that activity. You can feel Ikigai when you have coffee in the morning, you can feel Ikigai when you work in the garden, and you can feel Ikigai when you watch heart-warming movies.

If people ask you what your Ikigai is, in this case, you can say morning coffee is my Ikigai, gardening is my Ikigai, or watching heart-warming movies is my Ikigai.

Another meaning of Ikigai is a life purpose or a reason for living. This is more relevant if you have a mission in your life. For example, I want to create a world where everyone is happy. That is my mission in life, and I feel I was born for that. Everything I have been doing in my life so far contributes to that goal in one way or another. Now I want to accomplish it through spreading the Ikigai Diet.

Therefore, spreading the Ikigai Diet is my Ikigai now. It happens to be my job, too, in my case, but it doesn't have to be a job, it could be any kind of mission.

By the way, have you seen the framework of four interlocking circles that form a Venn diagram? There are the following keywords in each circle.

1. What you love

2. What you are good at
3. What the world needs
4. What you can be paid for

In the center of the circles, there is a word Ikigai.

Many people seem to associate Ikigai with this framework, but it is not a concept in Japan. It is spreading only outside of Japan, and most Japanese people haven't seen it. It doesn't represent the meaning of the Japanese word Ikigai. Ikigai is just a word, and it isn't a framework or a self-improvement method.

If you want to find your life mission, I suppose you can apply the first three keywords, but not the last one, unless you want to make your life mission a job.

This concept applies more if you want to find an Ikigai business, a business with your life mission. Actually, I wrote another book called *IKIGAI BUSINESS: The Secret of Japanese Omi Merchants to Find a Profitable, Meaningful, and Socially Friendly Business*. It is based on Omi-merchants' concept of Sanpo-Yoshi, and it isn't directly related to this Ikigai framework, but it applies to it, too.

## HAVING A LIFE MISSION

As I said before, Ikigai has two meanings.

1. A small joy in daily life
2. A life purpose or a reason for living

Ikigai as a small joy in daily life is good for your well-being since it gives you something to look forward to each day, and quite often, it is regarded as valuable in retirement life. To lead a happy retirement life, it is good to have a hobby or some kind of daily pleasure.

Many things I have introduced in this book can be your Ikigai; Nordic walking, gardening, yoga, and mountain hiking.

However, to lead a truly fulfilling life, you want to have more than that. You want to have Ikigai as your life mission.

Well, why do you want to live long in the first place? If there is no purpose in life, there isn't much point in extending your life until age 100, is there? We might as well die in our 80s as most people have been doing.
Why do we live anyway? What is the purpose of our life? We need to ask ourselves this ultimate question when we pursue the quest for longevity.

If you have some kind of spiritual belief, it is easier to have a life mission based on your belief, and the fact that many people in Blue Zones have some form of faith shows that having a life purpose can help your longevity more.

In that case, is it better to have a religion?

In many ways, it seems to help if you believe in something. You feel more elevated if you live your life based on higher callings. Nevertheless, you don't have to be religious in the traditional sense to have a life purpose. We all want to be happy, don't we? We all want to live in a happy society, too, because in order to be truly content, we want our family and friends to be happy, as well as the wider social community. In other words, you want to live in a Sanpo-Yoshi society.

## BUILDING A SANPO-YOSHI SOCIETY AS YOUR LIFE MISSION

I told you that my mission in life was to create a world where everyone is happy, and this can be your life mission, too. One person alone cannot build a utopia, it can only be accomplished by the collective efforts of many people. If you have your own spiritual practice, that's fine, you can have your Ikigai based on that, but if you don't have one, making the world happier can be your Ikigai. It is a new spirituality among Shizenha people in Japanese Satoyama. Some of them are spiritual in the sense that they practice yoga, Taoism, or Shinto, but many people don't necessarily believe in higher beings. Yet, they live based on love: Love of humanity and Mother Earth. They respect one another and value diversity.

## WAYS TO BUILD A SANPO-YOSHI SOCIETY

You can promote organic farming to create a happy society. Supporting alternative medicine is another way. Enhancing economic localization is another. You can work toward gender equality or racial and cultural tolerance. You can also work to decrease the gap between rich and poor. There are many different ways to make the world better.

## Do What You Love

Although I said that the Ikigai framework of Venn diagram didn't represent the Japanese word Ikigai, two of the keywords in the framework can be useful to find your mission, You can think of what you love doing in some of those fields. I chose writing because that is what I love to do the most. I get so much pleasure out of writing. I write books along with these themes.

## Do What You are Good At

I am spreading a diet that is based on the Japanese dietary culture to the world because I am in a position where I can easily do it, being Japanese, staying young and healthy myself, and speaking English. If you choose a field you have some expertise in, you are more likely to be able to give value to society.

## The Ikigai Diet Can be Your Ikigai

If you can't find your Ikigai as a life mission, don't worry about it. Practicing the Ikigai Diet itself can be your mission. It is designed as a Sanpo-Yoshi diet. By following this diet, you will be happy, your family and friends will be happy, and society will be happy.

Think about it. How many people you know suffer from cancer, diabetes, or dementia because of their diet and lifestyle? A lot comes from social conditioning. The culture led by big corporations encourages us to consume fast food, meat-based dishes, and sugar-filled products. These corporations operate based on the philosophy of Urite-Yoshi, the seller is happy, and don't care about buyers and society. With cutting edge advertisements based on human psychology, they entice us to damage ourselves.

Do you want to let it keep happening? By practicing the Ikigai Diet, you will be an example for people around you. You can be a positive influencer. You might reach just one or two persons, but that's okay, because they might affect their family and friends. Gradually, this movement will grow. If you enjoy the diet, it will magnetize people automatically. All you need to do is to form a social circle of family and friends and support one another's wellness. You don't need to go out on the street to protest or put you on a strict diet. You can just have fun with your life.

## Satoyama Life Can be Your Ikigai

If you move to the countryside and lead a Satoyama lifestyle, you can easily find your Ikigai, too. Everything in Satoyama can be a new discovery or joy; growing vegetables in your garden, taking a walk in the woods, and cooking on wildfire. You can lead a sustainable lifestyle more easily in the countryside since you can be more self-sufficient. You can also support the local economy and encourage economic localization. Many thinkers such as Helena Norberg-Hodge and Satish Kumar believe that a lot of the world's problems like wars and climate change are caused by economic globalization, and we need to shift to localization. It is easier to localize our economy if many of us move to the countryside from big cities. Therefore by living in the countryside you are part of the change, and it is a socially friendly lifestyle.

## The Ikigai Diet Helps You Fulfill Your Mission

I decided to call this diet the Ikigai Diet because having Ikigai along with a healthy diet is crucial to your well-being and longevity, but also, this diet helps you live based on your Ikigai.

Having a life mission is critical, but what is more vital is fulfilling your mission. However, many of us drift away from our course after a while. We get caught up with our daily events and forget about our mission. One of the reasons why we can't stay on track, I think, is that we are not in balance. Our physical and mental conditions are not in balance, and we can't stay in tune with our source. A lot comes from our diet. What you eat and how you eat influences your state. How you use your brain, too. Therefore in the Ikigai Diet, we provide a holistic framework to work on your body, mind, and spirit all at the same time so that you can continue to be in tune with your source.

It is a diet to help you lead a long healthy life, but the ultimate goal of the Ikigai Diet is to help you stay focused on your life mission.

## LIVE WITH PASSION & MEANING

Longevity is our goal, but there isn't much point in having a long life if that is the only thing a person does. What will happen if this diet can help many of you, both young and old, find your Ikigai as your life mission and stay with your Ikigai? You will live with joy and passion every day. You will get up every morning full of energy, wanting to change the world to be a happy place. You will be grateful for everything you do. And you will think of your happiness, your family members' and friends' happiness, as well as your society's happiness. By the time you reach 100, which I am sure you will, the world will have become a utopia.

## FINAL SUMMARY

Now, let me sum up what I have covered in this book.

1. Use organically or naturally grown ingredients.

2. Use locally grown ingredients.

3. Eat and make fermented foods.

4. Eat whole food, Ma Go Wa Ya Sa Shi I, dietary fiber, and One Soup Three Dishes.

5. Not all carbs are bad for you; you don't need to avoid whole grains.

6. Eat fermented brown rice, wheat berries, oat groats, barley groats, and other grains.

7. Eat local cuisines.

8. Avoid consuming soft drinks, sweets, French fries, chips, other snacks, processed food, fruit juice, meat, and dairy products.

9. When you eat, eat vegetables first, then protein, and finally, carbs.

10. Stop eating when you are 80% full, chew a lot, don't eat between meals, or skip breakfast to give your gut plenty of breaks.

11. Drink a lot of water.

12. Don't become too strict about your diet and enjoy eating.

13. Use Hare and Ke to balance your diet.

14. Bring hygge and Zen into your dinner and make your eating a cozy and sacred experience.

15. Make exceptions when you socialize with others or eat out.

16. Create a social circle that can influence one another positively.

17. The Ikigai Diet isn't just a diet; it is a lifestyle, including exercises and mindset.

18. Find a suitable exercise such as walking or Nordic walking and do it daily.

19. Train your internal organs instead of your muscles.

20. You want to build flexible muscles rather than big muscles.

21. Think positive.

22. Past successful experience meditation.

23. Shinon Kansha and be grateful for what is happening in your life.

24. Move to the countryside and practice a Satoyama lifestyle.

25. Find Ikigai as your life mission.

26. Working toward building a Sanpo-Yoshi society can be your life mission.

27. You can find your Ikigai through what you love doing.

28. You can find your Ikigai through what you are good at.

29. The Ikigai Diet can be your Ikigai.

30. Satoyama life can be your Ikigai.

31. Fulfill your life's mission.

Well, thank you very much for reading this book. I hope you got something out of it. I know we have covered a lot of things. It takes time to incorporate all of this into your cooking. Just start applying these strategies in your life one by one. Once you get used to practicing one menu, you can move on to the next one.

I would love to have some feedback from you. I would appreciate it very much if you left a review on the Amazon book page. I look forward to hearing from you.

Good luck on your journey toward wellness.


For more information, check out the following website.

The Ikigai Diet
https://ikigaidiet.com/

Here, I cover topics such as fermented food, organic food, autophagy, intermittent fasting, Japanese natural food movement, organic farming, Ikigai exercises, Satoyama living, and Ikigai mindset. I am especially interested in sharing current Japanese trends in health and well-being that are not shared much abroad since many books and magazine articles dealing with these topics are not written in English.

## ZEN AND A WAY OF SUSTAINABLE PROSPERITY

This is an e- book I wrote. *Zen and a Way of Sustainable Prosperity: A Teaching of Omi Merchants Who Thrived In 18th Century Japan.* This is a book to help you become sustainably prosperous, but in many ways, it contains clues to build a Sanpo-Yoshi society.

Chapter 1: A Fatal Flaw I Discovered in Motivational Success Philosophies
Chapter 2: Why Did I Get a Mansion from an Omi Merchant for Almost Free?
Chapter 3: The Secret of Omi-Merchants' Business Success
Chapter 4: Business Model of Making Society Happy
Chapter 5: The 7 Elements of Sustainable Prosperity
Chapter 6: Choosing a Business that Has the Element of Three-Way Satisfaction
Chapter 7: Yin and Yang of Goal Setting
Chapter 8: How to Plan Your Success with the Method of Natural Farming
Chapter 9: Unleashing the Magic Number 33 to Align Yourself with Success
Chapter 10: The Key to Success is Measuring Your Progress and Customizing Your Method
Chapter 11: The Right and Wrong Way of Using the Law of Attraction
Chapter 12: The Key to Manifestation is Successfully Dealing with Your Past Experiences
Chapter 13: How to Have a Positive Relationship with Money
Chapter 14: Zen Meditation Can Set You in the Right Mood to Start Your Day
Chapter 15: Healthy Intestines are the New Symbols of Success
Chapter 16: Enlightenment is the Ultimate Key to Prosperity

*Zen and a Way of Sustainable Prosperity. A Teaching of Omi Merchants Who Thrived In 18th Century Japan*
https://www.amazon.com/dp/B072LBFFYS/

**IKIGAI BUSINESS**

If you are interested in shifting your lifestyle and changing your job, you might find it useful to read another e-book I wrote *IKIGAI BUSINESS: The Secret of Japanese Omi Merchants to Find a Profitable, Meaningful, and Socially Friendly Business.*

Table of Contents

*IKIGAI BUSINESS: The Secret of Japanese Omi Merchants to Find a Profitable, Meaningful, and Socially Friendly Business*
https://www.amazon.com/dp/B079Z24B1Z

## ABOUT THE AUTHOR

Sachiaki Takamiya is a writer and the founder of the Ikigai Diet. As a writer, he has written many books. His best-known work is a spiritual adventure novel called *Tenjo-no-Symphony*, which was published in Japanese from Kodansha in 2006. In English, he has written *Zen and a Way of Sustainable Prosperity*, and *IKIGAI BUSINESS*.

He lived in England in his early 20s, where he studied Shiatsu and macrobiotics at the British School of Shiatsu, studied different kinds of psychotherapies at the Center for Counselling and Psychotherapy Education and at the School of Hypnosis and Advanced Psychotherapy.

After returning to Japan, he began giving workshops on holistic transformation based on his studies of both physical and psychological approaches.

He now lives in a small rural town called Hino town in Shiga Prefecture, which is one of the longest-lived prefectures in Japan. He practices a Satoyama lifestyle there, growing vegetables and making fermented foods. Although he will be 60 years old this year, he hasn't had any problems at medical check-ups so far, and he was diagnosed that his vascular age was 21 years younger.

He also has a network of naturalist friends in Hino Town, surrounding areas in Shiga Prefecture, and all over Japan.

The Ikigai Diet
https://ikigaidiet.com/

The Ikigai Diet YouTube channel
https://www.youtube.com/channel/UCITxFTF4x1lgdh0vLKXC- CAw

The Ikigai Diet and Bio-Hacking Newsletter
https://landing.mailerlite.com/webforms/landing/i4x0r3https://landing.mail erlite.com/webfor...

The Ikigai Diet: The Secret Japanese Diet to Health and Longevity
Written by Sachiaki Takamiya
Published by Zen Quest on September 22nd, 2020
The second edition on May 28th, 2021
Zen Quest http://www.zenquest.net/
ISBN 978-4-9910648-6-9

Made in the USA
Coppell, TX
20 February 2024

29222164R00067